T0353778

Eat TROPICAL

To HEAL

A Guide To Preventing And Reversing Obesity, Cardiovascular Diseases and type 2 Diabetes with Tropical Foods and the SET-FREE method.

By

MARLYSE L. K. ASSONKEN-SOBTAFO

Balboa Press books may be ordered through booksellers or by contacting:

Balboa Press
A Division of Hay House
1663 Liberty Drive
Bloomington, IN 47403
www.balboapress.com
844-682-1282

ISBN: 979-8-7652-5418-9 (sc)
979-8-7652-5417-2 (e)

Library of Congress Control Number: 2024915724

Print information available on the last page.

Balboa Press rev. date: 08/21/2024

BALBOA.PRESS
A DIVISION OF HAY HOUSE

Table of Contents

Acknowledgment:

I want to express my heartfelt gratitude to everyone who offered feedback on my book during its early stages. Special thanks go to my husband, Dr. Cyriaque Sobtafo, for his unwavering support throughout this project. I am also deeply appreciative of my baby sister, Dr. Francine Assonken-Atte, for her invaluable medical insights. My heartfelt thanks go to the head of my children's crew, Landry Sobtafo, for his fresh perspective and valuable feedback, and to Cindy Sobtafo, the youngest of the crew and the artist who designed the book cover and took some of the pictures. To each of my children from Landry, Karen, Jordan to Cindy, for their enduring presence and encouragement.

I must also express my gratitude to my father, Benoit Assonken, and my brothers, Yannick, Ronny, Blondel, Patrick, and their spouses for their steadfast support. Martine Inack-Thieulin, your daily interactions, friendship, generosity, and feedback have inspired me greatly. Olga Korobova Vasseur, your support, friendship, and inspiration have been invaluable. My thanks also extend to my in-laws for their backing.

Further appreciation goes to Jude Nguimfack Tsague and Jean Kironde for their insightful feedback.

Lastly, I want to give a huge shoutout to "Family Meeting," a Cameroonian association based in Dakar that I am part of. Thank you for your collective effort in making my book publishing dream a reality.

Special thanks are also due to everyone around the world who agreed to share brief testimonials of your health outcomes following the nutritional and lifestyle support I provided. I have intentionally used pseudonyms in my book to maintain your anonymity and protect your privacy.

Dedication

This book is dedicated to my mom,
who lost her life to T2D and cardiovascular diseases. Je t'aime maman.

Introduction

In a world influenced by Western culture, the dominance of the Western diet is evident. Unfortunately, tropical countries in Africa, Pacific Islands, and the Caribbean, often less developed and more vulnerable, tend to adopt this trend without realizing the hidden potential of their local foods.

This book aims to redirect attention to the healing power of local foods in tropical regions, shedding light on their often-overlooked benefits. It is on a mission to change how we think about food and health. Instead of blindly following Western diets, the book uncovers the incredible healing powers of tropical local foods. But it's not just about what you eat—it's also about taking control of your own health. The goal is to empower you with the tools and knowledge to be your own healthcare hero.

If you're struggling with conditions like obesity, Type 2 Diabetes, or heart disease, there's hope. This book shows that these conditions aren't set in stone – they can be reversed.

At the heart of it all is the SET-FREE method, a robust framework I crafted from years of experience, grounded in science, and enriched by insights from health experts, ancient traditional food, and wellness practices. It's more than just physical health—it's also about nurturing mental well-being and finding balance in your life. With four pillars to steer you, this book provides a comprehensive guide that serves as your pathway to a healthier, happier you.

So, what does SET-FREE stand for?

SET - SEASONAL AND TRADITIONAL FOOD:

Enjoy the wholesome benefits of whole, seasonal, and minimally processed local foods.

F - FASTING:

Discover how intermittent fasting can be a game-changer.

RE - ROUTINE EXERCISE:

Discover the different ways regular exercise can benefit you.

E - BE THE EXPERT ON YOUR HEALTH:

Take charge of your well-being and be your own doctor to transform your body and mind.

This holistic health approach serves as a compass for not just a healthy diet but also for keeping active, growing personally, and maintaining a sound mind. I bring a wealth of experience as a functional nutritionist, and my time as a radio commentator diving into personal development issues has added another layer of insight. But that's not all – I'm also a passionate 2nd Dan black belt in Taekwondo, a long-distance runner, and an all-around sports enthusiast. That passion for sport is woven into the fabric of what you'll find in these pages. It's not just expertise; it's a real-world guide to your health journey!

You are invited to explore an approach that puts you front and center in your health journey, aiming to help you achieve long-lasting health and happiness.

Stay with me, and I'll help you every step of the way. But wait, there's more! I'll also share recipes and tips as the icing on the cake to make this adventure more empowering!

Monique:

Since I started fasting and using the SET-FREE method, my sleep has drastically improved. I wake up feeling truly rested, and my mornings kick off with a newfound clarity and creativity. I am more performant at work. The weight loss has been a welcomed bonus, but the real surprise has been the peace of mind I've discovered on this journey of letting go. Fasting became a catalyst for releasing control. The only challenge? Navigating the restart of eating without feeling the need to catch up. For me, the most formidable aspect of fasting isn't the hunger; it's the persistent images of food playing in my mind.

Chapter 1:

Nutrition and Lifestyle Fall Apart In Africa, The Caribbean And The Pacific

I have traveled and lived all around the world, and embarking on a global journey opened my eyes to the incredible diversity of our planet. Living in different countries on various continents was not just cool—it was an eye-opener. I immersed myself in Western, African, Pacific, and Asian cultures, soaking up the unique ways people live.

This adventure became a vital lesson on how lifestyle choices impact our health. With over 15 years of experience in hospitals, private practice, and international organizations, I've encountered clients and patients worldwide. What struck me is the growing stress in people's lives and the shift away from traditional, wholesome foods.

In today's fast-paced world, many are reaching for sugary and deep-fried delights instead of real, nourishing food. Take a moment to ponder the sugar content in your daily intake—did you know a single can of soda packs in more than ten teaspoons of sugar? It's like an instant immune system disruptor!

Water, once the universal go-to, seems to be losing its charm. Even the refreshing allure of coconut water often gets overshadowed by the tempting pull of soda, which has become the default choice thanks to aggressive promotion on social media, eye-catching posters, and its availability around every corner. This shift in our drinking and eating habits is altering our taste buds and impacting our overall well-being.

As I traveled, I couldn't help but notice the changing landscape of how we move around. Take Fiji, for example. You can ask the bus to halt wherever you please; it's a pretty handy perk. However, what caught my attention was the clever strategy of hopping off just seconds after the last stop, avoiding any unnecessary strolls.

Transportation has evolved into a myriad of options in Africa. Cars and buses are king, and motorcycles rule the road. In Uganda and Kenya, it's the trusty *Boda Boda*[1], in Cameroon, the

---

[1] Boda boda, Bensikin and Okada are bicycles or motorcycles used as a taxi for carrying a passenger or goods.

Bensikin, and in Nigeria, the ever-popular *Okada*. These rides don't just get you close to your destination; they practically drop you at the doorstep.

It's common to witness motorcycle acrobatics, with riders skillfully balancing five to six passengers spread around them. Some creative owners even tweak their bikes, adding extra seats to meet the high demand. It's a wild ride, quite literally! The struggle for balance becomes part of the adventure, but in the end, everyone's smiling. Customers save time (if they arrive safely), and the motorcyclist pockets some extra cash. It's a win-win, albeit with a dash of thrilling chaos! Walking is losing its appeal, even for short distances like a nearby store or the neighbor's house.

As a nutritionist, I've witnessed firsthand how our modern way of living is taking a toll on people's health. It's disheartening to see friends, family, and even colleagues unknowingly fall into the trap of believing this contemporary lifestyle is the only path forward. Little do they realize that their approach to modernity might be the root cause of their physical and mental health challenges.

Data from various countries reinforces the link between a poor lifestyle and unhealthy eating habits as the primary culprits behind the rising rates of obesity, Type 2 Diabetes, cardiovascular diseases, some types of cancer, and other preventable diseases. This concern is particularly significant in regions like Africa, the Pacific, and the Caribbean. The good news? We have the power to change it, and that's the main focus of my book.

1. Modernization: How Africans, The Caribbean, And The Pacific Islanders handle it against Their Well-Being

Picture this: A lively scene in tropical countries where the beat of progress and the marvels of new technology join forces in an exhilarating dance. It's like setting off on an adventure filled with the promise of a more comfortable life. But wait, if you zoom in a bit, there are a few stumbling blocks amidst the dazzling lights.

The call for modernization is like a charming whisper to these nations, urging them to swap some cherished traditions for the sleek trends of the West. This trend gained momentum post-independence, but it's been a rapid and somewhat unplanned journey that has impacted the people's well-being.

Imagine trying to solve a puzzle—we're on a quest to discover that perfect balance between the glitzy modern lifestyle and the reliable, healthier traditions we hold dear. The whirlwind of technological progress spins so fast around us, leaving little time to pause and ponder. In this constant rush, we might not even notice the subtle toll it's taking on our health, each impulsive action chipping away at our well-being.

Consider how we get around these days. Convenience takes the spotlight, and choosing to walk might raise some eyebrows. But here's the scoop – physical activity is our health hero. It's vital. So, picture it as a graceful dance, where we navigate the swift modern world while still embracing the age-old wisdom of healthier living. It's a bit like a balancing act, resembling the rumba—an Afro-Cuban waltz—we're dancing to this well-being journey together.

Now, shifting gears to food–quick and easy options like fast food and processed goodies are gaining popularity because who wants to spend hours in the kitchen, right? Walk into a grocery store, and you'll find shelves filled with vegetable oil, canned goods, white rice, pasta, cookies, sugary drinks, chips, and more. Even street vendors lure us in with tempting fried delights like *Puff puffs*[2], samosas, *Akara,* and *Kabalagala*. These tasty treats, however, can pave the way for health issues, yet we often make them our go-to snacks. It's time for a little rethink, don't you think?

Outside food and exercise, well-being also encompasses mental health. Let me take you back to when I first moved to Canada, making it my new home. Surrounded by family and friends, they were super helpful and caring. They were primarily concerned about practical things like where I'd live and whether I had a car or a job. Yet, we rarely dug into how I felt inside, handling all these changes. We seldom explored those non-material aspects that go beyond money or physical things. It's the way we've been wired to think, and truth be told, it often leads us to sideline our emotional well-being, a crucial factor for our happiness.

In the hustle and bustle of modern life, there's a strong emphasis on making money and accumulating stuff. People tend to gauge their value by possessions and constantly compare themselves to others. It seems like everyone's yearning for a sleek car, a cozy house, or the latest iPhone or Samsung gadget. Technology evolves rapidly, and the pressure to keep up drives us to work more, often in competitive and stressful environments. In this pursuit, our well-being takes a back seat, as long as we earn enough to buy these coveted things. It turns into a cycle where we splurge on possessions but cut corners on our health and happiness. We end up having plenty of possessions but little time to enjoy our wealth, do things we love or spend quality time with loved ones.

This relentless cycle impacts our mental and physical health; it's likely you know someone—a family member, neighbor, or a friend's family—struggling with issues like persistent sadness or depression, anger management issues, excess weight, or other health problems rooted in their lifestyle.

---

[2]   Puff Puffs (West Africa), also known as Mandazi (East Africa), *Amagwinya (south Africa)* are beloved snacks made from deep fried dough scooped and cut into round shapes. They are made with a blend of wheat flour, sugar, salt, yeast, and water. Some people may choose to enhance the recipe with additional ingredients such as butter or eggs.

Akara is a Sub-saharan snack made by mixing black-eyed bean paste with salt and spices, scooped with a spoon, and then deep-fried.

Kabalagala is a Sub-Saharan snack made by mixing cassava paste with ripe banana and sugar, then scooped with a spoon and then deep-fried.

Here's the real deal: We create more than one harmful cycle. We also set up and actively feed what I like to call the "Modern Lifestyle Drama Triangle," which I'll unravel in the next chapter.

" Man sacrifices his health to make money. Then he sacrifices money to recuperate his health. And then, he is so anxious about the future that he does not enjoy the present; the result is that he does not live in the present or the future. He lives as if he is never going to die, then dies having never really lived."

Dalai Lama

2. Modern Lifestyle Drama Triangle: The Sugar Addition, Eating Frequency, Insulin Dilemma, and Disease Connection

In this section, I'll break down how we've become trapped in a modern lifestyle cycle dominated by added sugar, frequent eating, and chronic stress. These are the main non-medical factors that disrupt our insulin production, leading to chronic health issues. Our addiction to certain foods and harmful habits keeps us trapped in this loop. Unfortunately, we often pass these behaviors down to our children, creating a "Modern Lifestyle Drama Triangle" (depicted in Figure1) that affects multiple generations.

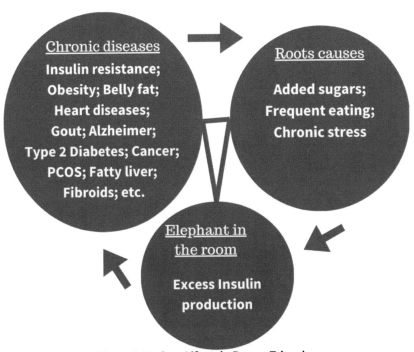

Figure 1: Modern Lifestyle Drama Triangle

Note: PCOS stands for Polycystic Ovary Syndrome. PCOS is a condition where women produce a lot of male hormones. This can result in irregular periods, extra hair on the face or body, and more insulin produced, which can cause weight gain, especially around the belly. Those symptoms typically become apparent during the late teenage years.

I'll break down each part of this triangle, starting with added sugars, then moving on to the impact of a stressful lifestyle, and finally frequent eating. I'll explore how each of these root causes influences insulin levels and, in turn, affects our overall health.

2.1. Added Sugar Invasion: Effects on Insulin and Health

Added Sugar Invasion

Our food world is naturally sweet, with sugars in fruits, tubers, grains, coconut water, and milk. What makes these sugars unique is that they come with built-in 'sugar damage control,' like fibers, fats, proteins, and antioxidants—a complete package that our bodies are designed to handle. Unlike the sugars we find in processed foods, the sugars in traditional foods don't send our insulin levels on a rollercoaster ride.

Now, let's talk about what I call the "added sugar invasion." It's a widespread trend where sugar and syrups sneak into almost everything we eat and drink, whether it's store-bought or homemade. This intense sweetness has become a staple in processed foods, and we've become so accustomed to it that we're even sprinkling sugar into dishes we prepare ourselves. Picture this: *Yassa sauce* with onion and mustard, *Sanga* with amaranth leaves or cassava leaves with corn, and the local favorites like Bissap or sorrel, baobab, and ginger juices—all getting a generous dose of sugar.

And it doesn't stop there. We've welcomed sugar into our daily rituals, adding it to our coffee, tea, and desserts. It's like we've declared a sweet takeover in our kitchens and dining tables. But, as we indulge in these sweet moments, it's crucial to be mindful of the impact of excessive added sugar on our health. We can savor the natural sweetness of whole foods and strike a balance in our sugar adventures.

Tropical countries worldwide boast a treasure trove of delectable sweet snacks that are delightful and easily accessible from the friendly neighborhood street vendor. Each Tropical region has unique treats, from the mouthwatering Deep-fried snacks to the tempting caramelized nuts and seeds.

Venturing into the Caribbean, you'll discover delightful desserts like *Cassava Pone* and *Rhum Cake*. *Cassava Pone*, a Caribbean delicacy, blends grated cassava roots with coconut, milk, sugars, and spices, creating a heavenly cake baked to golden-dark perfection. It's a flavor explosion that mirrors the creativity of other sugary snacks and desserts across the Caribbean.

In Fiji, *Bila* and *Ivi* take center stage as beloved sweet snacks. *Bila*, a wrapped and steamed delight, involves fermented cassava cooked in banana leaves, with an extra sprinkle of Fijian sugar magic. *Ivi*, on the other hand, features ground chestnut baked in banana leaves, sweetened to perfection. Even fresh fruits get a sugary makeover in Fiji, as they add syrup to enhance their natural sweetness.

Added sugars come with many different names. Some you might know, like brown and white sugar, cane juice, corn syrup, agave syrup, maple syrup, and raw sugar. Others that sound fancy and are hidden behind names such as dextrose, fructose, fruit nectars, glucose, high-fructose corn syrup, lactose, malt syrup, maltose, molasses, sucrose, corn sweeteners, hydrolyzed starch, inverted sugar, palm syrup, and rice syrup.

Now, I bet you're curious about the wonders of honey. It turns out that pure honey, in reasonable amounts (it's a sugar after all!), is fantastic for blood sugar! While the exact magic behind its blood sugar benefits is still a bit mysterious, pure honey has this incredible ability to lower high blood sugar levels. It's also used for several other medicinal purposes in small amounts and for a limited period. However, when honey is mixed with sugars for commercial reasons, it can become a health hiccup, behaving just like those regular sugars we try to avoid. So, the golden rule is to know your honey – opt for the pure kind to enjoy the sweet benefits in moderation, without the sugar shenanigans.

Not all added sugars are the same; they contain varying amounts of fructose and glucose, impacting our bodies differently. I'll delve into the details in the next section, but before we get there, check out the percentages of fructose and glucose in some common added sugars summarized in Table 1 below. I'll also walk you through their distinctive characteristics.

Table 1: Proportions of fructose and glucose in added sugars

Added Sugars	Characteristics	Glucose	Fructose
Table sugar (sucrose)	Once we extract juice from sugar cane, we purify and filter it to create golden, raw sugar, which is then turned into the table sugar we use.	50%	50%
Agave syrup	After extracting the juice from the agave plant sap, we filter, heat, and concentrate it into a syrup. Agave is known for its very high fructose content.	20%	80%
Marple syrup	Natural sweetener obtained from the sap of maple tree	48%	42%
Coconut sugar	Coconut sugar comes from the sap of the coconut palm. This sap circulates through the tree in a similar way to maple syrup.	35-40%	35-40%

High Fructose Corn Syrup (HFCS)	HFCS is processed from cheap corn, making it a cheaper sugar industry uses to enhance the taste of processed food and sweetened beverages. Manufacturers add HFCS to several processed foods, including fast foods, ketchup, breakfast cereals, sodas, bread, baked goods, sweetened milk, and candies.	45%	55%

If you have a sweet tooth, check this out! Table 1 makes it pretty clear: agave and HFCS are like sugar twins. They both contain a lot of fructose.

But why should we care about fructose? Here's why: Fructose, a sugar found in higher amounts in agave and friends (see Table 1), is a troublemaker for our bodies. It's like the mischief-maker compared to its counterpart, glucose.

So, buckle up, sugar explorers! I am about to unravel the secrets of fructose and glucose – because knowing the difference might just be the key to keeping our sweet cravings in check.

The Impact of Glucose and Fructose on Insulin Levels and Disease

Ever wondered how much-added sugar is too much? According to the Dietary Guidelines for Americans, adults shouldn't have more than 200 calories from added sugar daily. That's like 10-12 teaspoons of sugar, the same as in one can of soda or what you might add to a mug of local drinks like *Bissap*, the hibiscus leaves, or ginger juice. If someone drinks one or two cans of sodas or the same amount of local juice, they might already be going over the recommended sugar limit for the day. And that's just from drinks. Sugar can add up even more if we eat processed foods.

Watch out for the hidden "virus" in the sugary delights—a sweetness invasion passed down through generations. This sugar "virus" can create added sugar addiction and lead to a cascade of health issues. It's a concern reflected in the health landscape, as illustrated in Figure 1. So, while enjoying the delightful treats, let's also be mindful of our sugar intake and savor these indulgences in moderation.

Interestingly, we often hear about how glucose can impact our health by increasing insulin levels. But we don't usually think about what fructose does. It wasn't until 2004 that Dr. George Bray from Louisiana State University explained how fructose can make us gain weight and was even the main culprit of the obesity problem. That's when people began to notice and care more about this sugar.

Similarities Between Glucose And Fructose

So, consuming excessive amounts of fructose and glucose, make us age faster. These sugars harm our DNA, disrupt cell metabolism, and mess with our body's ability to repair. As a result, our cells become more vulnerable to conditions like cancer, Alzheimer's, cardiovascular diseases, and type 2 diabetes. As a result, our cells become more vulnerable to conditions like cancer, Alzheimer's, cardiovascular diseases, and type 2 diabetes, as shown in Figure 1 above. Additionally, they impact our skin, causing it to lose its glow and potentially increasing facial hair. Oh, and watch out for fructose especially—it's like the heavyweight champion of DNA damage, potentially making us age up to seven times faster than glucose.

Differences Between Glucose And Fructose

Glucose is like a good friend who can turn into a troublemaker, while fructose is more like a silent killer. Here's why:

Fructose doesn't make us feel full. Companies use a type of sugar called HFCS, made from cheap corn, to make processed foods tastier and kind of addictive. You can find HFCS in fast food, soda, packaged drinks, ketchup, bread, crackers, snacks, candies, salad dressings, canned foods, and more. The crazy thing is, these sugary foods are designed to keep us coming back for more. Plus, they become our go-to comfort food, boosting our mood when we're stressed, anxious, or down. It's like a quick fix that makes us feel happy, similar to how a drug addict gets that shot to escape life's challenges for a moment.

Our bodies don't like fructose because our cells can't use it. Unlike glucose, fructose doesn't increase our blood sugar or give any warning signs. Instead, it quietly goes to our liver and turns into harmful fat. This fat can cause problems like belly fat, a fatty liver, high triglycerides, and bad cholesterol. It can even lower our good cholesterol. This fat can clog our arteries, leading to heart issues, and increase our risk of Type 2 Diabetes, gout, and other chronic conditions.

On the flip side, our bodies really like glucose, which all our cells, including the brain, use for energy. Glucose is a good kind of sugar that helps distribute our weight evenly. About 80% of the glucose from traditional grains and tubers we eat go to our body's cells, and only about 20% is stored in our liver as glycogen, which is a safe kind of sugar. This is why long-distance runners eat starchy foods to build up their glycogen stores for energy during a marathon. Only a tiny bit of glycogen may turn into fat. But having too much glucose can cause our sugar levels and insulin to spike and get disrupted.

Check Table 2 in the annex. It summarizes how different types of carbohydrates, from traditional foods to processed ones, affect our health.

Now that we understand more about the components of added sugar and how they affect insulin and our health, let's explore how eating too often can make us unwell, similar to adding sugar.

2.2. Eating Frequency: Effect On Insulin and Health

Eating Frequency

We're surrounded by a lot of food, especially fast and processed stuff, everywhere we look — on the streets, TV, posters, and social media. Avoiding the tempting food around us is tricky in today's world. We often eat not because we are hungry but because it is "mealtime." We eat numerous times in a day, probably too many to count. Eating has become like a habit – almost automatic, like a Pavlovian reflex, instead of a decision we make on purpose. How often have you heard someone say, "I'm hungry; let's have lunch"? Not very often, right? It's more like, "It's lunchtime, so let's eat." How frequently do we end up in the kitchen grabbing snacks like nuts, chips, fruit, or bread without really thinking about it? Sometimes, it's just out of boredom or stress. Even though these snacks might not feel like a proper meal, our bodies still react as if it is. Every meal is a task for our body to handle.

Eating Frequency, Insulin Levels, and Disease

Here's something important to understand: every time we eat, our insulin levels go up, and they stay up if we eat too often, no matter what kind of food it is. Even if we're eating healthy, traditional food, we can still make our insulin work too hard if we don't pay attention to when and how often we eat. When that happens, we enter the modern lifestyle drama triangle: our bodies store fat, gain weight, and are exposed to conditions described in Figure 1 above.

Stress, Insulin Levels, and Disease

Whenever we hear about stress, we usually just want to steer clear of it. But there are actually different kinds: acute stress, which can be beneficial, and chronic stress, which is the troublesome one.

Acute stress is the intense type that is supposed to happen occasionally. It is the healthier stress that stimulates our immune system and makes us more alert and focused to face the challenge. It makes us even more creative and boosts our motivation. Haven't you noticed how when we face danger we always push ourselves to where we never thought we could reach? In the process, we get out of our comfort zone to explore new ways to ultimately save our lives. That's the purpose of acute stress.

Over time, stress has become a constant companion in our lives, evolving way beyond what it was ever meant to be: it has become chronic. We've trapped ourselves in a never-ending loop of stress, driven by our own choices, unexpected events, and the actions of others. Whether it's someone crossing our boundaries, the fear of being judged, or the pressure to meet high expectations, stress always finds a way to creep in. And sometimes, just acknowledging how stressed we are adds even more stress, making it feel like an unavoidable part of life. The problems start when we reach this stage of chronic stress.

Chronic stress can mess with our emotions, making us feel more anxious, angry, sad, or irritable, and can even drain our motivation. It can also affect our behavior, leading to habits like smoking, skipping exercise, or overeating as a way to cope. Instead of finding relief, you might end up trapped in a loop of addiction to these habits.

Stress also causes the release of hormones like cortisol, known as the stress hormone. Cortisol and insulin are like close buddies—when cortisol levels stay high, it invites insulin to spike, leading to weight gain. This is why some people struggle to lose weight, even on a strict diet. As I discussed in Chapter 3, sections C and D, managing stress is crucial for keeping insulin levels stable and either avoiding or getting out of the Modern Lifestyle Drama Triangle.

2.3. Insulin: The Elephant In The Room of Our Health

So, basically, the thing messing up our health is insulin. It's super sensitive to added sugar and frequent eating. No matter what overstimulates insulin, it makes us sick in the same way. Insulin appears, therefore, to be the elephant in the room when it comes to our health. I'll dive deeper into insulin in the fasting chapter.

To sum it up, the modern lifestyle drama triangle kicks off with added sugar and frequent eating, then comes the insulin disruption, and finally, the cascade of health challenges.

So, imagine we're caught up in this drama triangle, like a cycle of problems. But guess what? I came up with a solution called the SET-FREE method. It's a practical plan that takes inspiration from how our ancestors ate and lived, but I've tweaked it to fit how we live today. Before I explain the details, I'll share in chapter two what made me create this method in the first place.

Amy :

My menopause belly has shrunk, and my libido has improved. Embracing the SET-FREE method has really worked wonders for me during menopause. It's amazing how a few positive changes can have such transformative effects on both body and mind!

Chapter 2:

Decoding The SET-FREE Method – My Journey From Unlearning to Crafting the SET-FREE Method

" Education is all about what you have unlearned."

Mark Twain

"Education is the most powerful weapon which you can use to change the world."

Nelson Mandela

In my job as a functional Nutritionist, I help people get healthier in two ways. One way is by working with the government to create big rules that affect everyone, like school nutrition programmes, national dietary guidelines and targeted nutrition programmes for specific vulnerable groups. But it takes a really long time to see results, and we're not sure if it works well for everyone. The other way is a more holistic care approach—I talk to individuals and help them one-on-one. I prefer this approach because I can really understand the whole picture of the person, and we can figure out their health issues together. For example, I once helped someone named Céline who wanted to lose weight. It turned out her real problem was feeling bad about herself, and that's why she ate for comfort. The big rules wouldn't have caught that, but with one-on-one talks, we could explore different aspects of her life and find a solution that worked for her. There are times when simply engaging in empathetic listening can make a significant difference.

However, not every case in my line of work has been a success. I remember an overweight client struggling with family health issues like diabetes, hypertension, and high cholesterol. Despite loving her ethnic food, she was super cautious with her diet, steering clear of red palm oil and starchy carbs, sticking mostly to veggies to keep her heart healthy and sugar levels steady. She was scared of her traditional food, and I wasn't well-prepared to guide her through it. This experience made me realize how little I knew about handling tropical food, opening up new questions and a fresh avenue for me to explore.

It was like breaking free from a metaphorical cage where I felt stuck doing things that didn't always sit right. I needed some fresh air to breathe and explore new paths. I had loads of questions about what I learned in university regarding food and health. I wanted to understand how diets changed over time, especially those ethnic diets that kept people healthy for ages. I wondered why some diets, like high-carb or high-fat, were labeled as bad when they've actually been keeping people healthy for a long time.

Take Africa, for instance, where Sahelian or Masai people eat a lot of meat without having more heart problems than the USA or the rest of the Western world. I was also curious about why red palm oil, groundnut oil, and coconut oil, which have been used for centuries, are now considered unhealthy. What harm did those oils do to our ancestors? Those folks were even more energetic and healthier than younger generations.

After digging into traditional diets worldwide and how they kept people healthy, I figured out there's no one-size-fits-all diet. Diets vary a lot based on where people live, their lifestyle, and their culture. But, the shared foundation for a healthy diet is consuming high-quality food, preferably directly from farms with minimal processing, regardless of your specific dietary approach.

This journey also led me to explore different ideas from experts, alternative medicine, and old traditions that have been keeping people healthy. That's where I discovered wellness practices from different parts of the world, like qigong in China, Yoga in India, and traditions in Africa, the Caribbean, and the Pacific. These practices believe in the amazing abilities of our bodies to take care of themselves, preventing and fixing illnesses for a long time. They primarily rely on traditional foods, incorporate fasting, meditate or pray, and maintain an active lifestyle.

In the West, the latest diet trends and superfoods take center stage, backed by billions of dollars in research. It's a big part of Western culture, tailored mainly for their population, to which they are responsible. However, in Tropical countries, there's significantly less research funding, and we often find ourselves merely following the Western food trends, which rarely align with our reality.

Keeping this Western food trend alive and in the spotlight requires pushing other foods aside. Guess which ones are the most vulnerable in this competition? Tropical foods. Our space has been taken over by unfair western criticism. Breaking this narrative is challenging because the West has way more resources; they control the funding and the media, shaping opinions to match their ideas. So, we often buy into their views, even when it comes to thinking our food is bad. In some West African countries, using palm oil is viewed as old-fashioned, and some folks even bleach red palm oil to make it seem less traditional, not realizing the potential harm it can cause.

On a related note, I've noticed a tendency where many people think doctors, nutritionists, and coaches will solve all their health problems. But actually, it's everyone's responsibility to stay healthy by making good choices every day. Health experts can help, but it's up to everyone to take care of themselves in their daily food and lifestyle decisions and choices.

Based on my experiences and observations working with clients from African, Caribbean, and Pacific countries, I re-evaluated my approach and identified some gaps. People in tropical regions often aren't aware of the healing power of their traditional foods, despite numerous studies supporting it. Many are still struggling to maintain the quality of their traditional diets in today's modern world. There's a strong focus on physical health, but true wellness goes beyond that, including emotional well-being, which is deeply connected to physical health.

This realization prompted me to step back for about a year and a half to explore new ideas and upgrade my approach. During that time, I cleaned up my knowledge about functional nutrition, tossed out the old stuff that wasn't working, and made room for fresh learning.

This meant staying open-minded, checking out different ways of thinking, diving into various studies, other healthcare providers' experience, and exploring ancient traditions that promote wellness. After all this, I came up with a method called the SET-FREE method, which I'll be talking about in chapter three. It's my way to help people in tropical countries stay healthy and heal, drawing on my expertise, new knowledge, and understanding their unique needs.

Anne:

For the past year, I've been following the SET-FREE method and practicing 16:8 and alternate-day fasting. The outcomes have been nothing short of amazing – not only did I witness significant weight loss, especially around my waist, but I also successfully brought my cholesterol and blood sugar levels back to the normal range. This program has truly been a game-changer for my overall health and well-being!

Chapter 3:

Unleashing the SET-FREE Method to Break the Vicious Cycle and Cultivate the Virtuous Cycle

I created the SET-FREE Method to help people stay healthy and heal, drawing on evidence-based information and my experiences working with individuals in hospitals and communities. I also checked out ancient traditional foods and wellness practices that prioritize not just physical health but also mental well-being and joy. This method is like a roadmap to break free from only hearing one side of the nutrition story pushed by the West. It's also about breaking free from thinking only doctors and therapists can keep you healthy. With SET-FREE, you take charge of your own health. It helps you change your health direction by figuring out, dealing with, and letting go of habits that aren't good for you. SET-FREE empowers you; the best part is that It doesn't cost anything. It gives you the tools and knowledge to be your own first doctor and lead your health journey.

The SET-FREE method is about four key things: (1) Traditional Food: I spill the beans on how awesome Tropical traditional food is. I talk about its healing power and how it triggers your five body defense mechanisms through various food types, traditional cooking methods, and food preservation tricks. (2) Fasting: In this section, I reveal how fasting is like having your personal health ally within. I'll walk you through the dos and don'ts of fasting, explore different fasting methods, and unveil the proven health benefits of incorporating fasting into your lifestyle. It's a guide to harnessing the power of fasting for your well-being (3) Regular Exercise: I dive into how exercise complements your nutrition, lifting both your body and mind; (4) Be Your First Doctor: Uncover the secrets to taking control of both your body and mind health. I dive into practical tips on caring for your mental well-being, just as you would for your physical health. It's a guide to nurturing both body and mind for a healthier, happier you. I share detailed knowledge and handy tools about these pillars. Get ready for the scoop!

A. Traditional Foods

The traditional food I'm delving into in this book is the real deal—whole food, the kind our ancestors enjoyed before colonization, modernization, and big industries changed our eating habits. This food mostly comes straight from farms and is minimally processed, featuring tubers (like cassava, yam, coco yams or *Dalo*, sweet potatoes or *kumara* or *Boniato*), proteins (such as fish, free-range chicken, grass-fed beef, beans, cowpeas, peas, lentils or dhal), and grains (like millet, sorghum, fonio, corn, and teff), along with veggies and fruits. Preservation back in the day didn't involve chemicals; instead, it embraced techniques like fermentation and drying. Unlike turning grains into white powder flour, they'd grind whole grains into nutritious flour using a stone or a mortar. As a quirky side note, I always carry a small grinding stone in my suitcases – it makes grinding spices easier and tastier. Traditional cooking might demand a bit more effort, but the incredible taste is the best reward.

Speaking of taste and tradition, let me take you back to the heartwarming memories of my childhood visits to Dschang, my village in Cameroon. One of the best parts was when my parents, siblings, and I visited my grandma, my father's mother. We usually started by Grandpa's house in the same compound before heading to her cozy room, surrounded by mud brick walls. As I approached, excitement filled the air—knowing I was about to see my grandmother. At the entrance, bamboo storage holds carefully selected dried grains ready to be planted for the next season. A warm, ashy, and spicy smell wrapped around me when I stepped inside, instantly making me feel at home.

In the room's heart, three stones with burning firewood supported a large pot filled with irresistible food, quietly simmering away. The taste was always a delight. A bamboo bed stood against the wall on one side, and underneath, special storage held cooked food for her favorite people. Several lines of corn on the cob dangled from the bamboo ceiling, beginning their drying journey. A bamboo ladder reached up to reveal the ceiling's hidden treasures—corn, beans, groundnuts, and other nuts completing their drying process.

As you glanced around, a unique corner held clay pots called *Nkan*, which, in my mother tongue, is a set of tools and mysterious items that add enchantment to the room. Even the mud floor seemed welcoming, making space for extra firewood just in case. I think the setup itself enhanced the flavor of the traditional food she cooked. Or maybe it was my grandmother's warm and generous personality, or her unique scent that added that special touch? The mystery remains, but one thing's for sure—I always left her place with a full belly and a happy heart.

1. The Healing Powers and Key Components of Tropical Traditional Foods

Traditional foods share a common thread, no matter where you are—they're a beacon of freshness, wholesomeness, and organic goodness. Picture this: fresh food from the farm, cows happily grazing on green pastures, and chickens freely pecking for their meals. It's a friendly team-up with nature, using very few chemicals, and everything is customized to match the environment's needs. It is all about quality!

But here's where the magic truly happens: traditional food is packed with nutrients. It's a powerhouse of goodness that satisfies your taste buds and contributes to preventing and curing diseases. And the excitement doesn't stop there—ongoing research keeps uncovering new antioxidants in these culinary wonders, adding an extra layer of health benefits.

More specifically, while many sing the praises of white meat, like chicken breast and wings, emerging knowledge highlights the goodness of dark meat, such as chicken thighs and drumsticks. Rich in vitamin K2, dark meat can potentially ward off cancer, improve heart health, and prevent arteries from hardening— we simply need to remove extra fat before consumption. It's great news for chicken drumstick enthusiasts, including my sons, brothers, and husband. Now, they can enjoy their favorite dark meat with the extra assurance that it brings some health benefits, contributing to a longer and healthier life.

Speaking of longevity, there are extraordinary places known as "blue zones" where people live the longest, including Loma Linda (USA), Okinawa (Japan), Nicoya (Costa Rica), Ikaria (Greece), and Sardinia (Italy). These locales are home to a significant number of centenarians! Their secret? It lies in traditional food and a lifestyle deeply rooted in strong community bonds. These places have yet to fully jump on the modern life bandwagon, highlighting how sticking to traditional practices can keep people healthy and living longer.

Now, as we dig into this idea of living longer, it's pretty interesting that the blue zones don't include tropical countries. But just because they're left out doesn't mean they can't be part of the story about living long lives. But think about it, who decided on those zones anyway? What if we created our own version focused on tropical areas and called it the 'black zone'? Sounds cool, right? It would finally put a positive spin on the tainted color. People in these "blue zones" areas are actually practicing habits that are common in many rural tropical communities as well. They grow their own food, eat mostly unprocessed produce, stay active, and keep strong ties with family and friends. Doesn't that sound just like life in many tropical villages? That's what I'm getting at!

Indeed, the strong sense of family and community support in African, Caribbean, and Pacific countries, particularly in rural areas less impacted by modernization, is a testament to the resilience of traditional values. Older folks in these regions often have a robust network of support, with relatives taking care of them. The community bonds run deep, providing a safety net for everyone through thick and thin. It's an amazing source of support for mental well-being. Yet, only a few of these groups can adapt to modern changes, especially keeping their traditional support systems alive.

what people eat largely depends on where they live, the weather, what's available, and their culture. Our bodies thrive with different foods in different environments. In hot areas like Africa, the Caribbean, and the Pacific, folks eat a lot of grains and tubers. Those carbs fill us up and release energy slowly, which is perfect when it's hot and we're active. It maintains a good level of energy over a long period. Additionally, sweating makes people lose water and salt, so the food might be a bit saltier in tropical places to compensate. Mother Nature even provides a naturally sweet drink option: coconut water. In tropical countries like Cote d'Ivoire, Pacific Islands, and Guyana, fresh coconut water is sold in the shell for a reasonable price. In places like Fiji, it seems like almost everyone has a coconut tree in their garden!

On islands or near the coast, the abundance of seafood becomes a cornerstone of the diet, complemented by the richness of coconut-based dishes and a foundation of carbohydrates. The ocean's bounty offers a variety of flavors and nutritional benefits.

On the other hand, inland communities like my village in Cameroon depend more on beans and various meats for protein. Before modernization brought fresh fish to every corner of the map, it wasn't common in my village. But, we found a smart workaround—dry fish. This not only adds a unique flavor to our local dishes but also highlights our community's creativity and resourcefulness in making sure everyone enjoys a delicious and well-rounded diet.

People living in the Sahel, where rains are very rare, eat a lot of millet and sorghum because these crops can grow even when it's hot and dry. Thus, their environment provides what their bodies need to stay healthy.

Nomadic tribes, like the Maasai in Kenya and Tanzania and the Fulani in West and Central Africa, eat a lot of meat, dairy, and butter from their animals. Some tribes, like those in Punjab, Gujarat, and Rajasthan in India, are mostly vegetarian.

Back in the day, folks in different societies didn't face much difficulty maintaining their weight. They rather had diverse body shapes shaped by their environments and lifestyles. Diets and lifestyles in each region were customized to people's needs, influencing how bodies developed to match their natural surroundings. For instance, the Sahelians and Maasai people used to be known for being slender. They didn't need a lot of physical strength but endurance because they herded animals and walked long distances. On the other hand, Bantou people are stocky and strong. They needed that strength for hunting, doing manual work, and surviving in their environment. Their bodies are prepared for challenges, like fighting ferocious animals such as lions. Even with lifestyle changes and mixing with other populations, those folks still carry those genes for their distinct body shape.

Now, let me tell you about my amazing dad. He used to be a star in football, and now he's in his 80s, still rocking it like a fit 40-year-old! His remarkable endurance and strength throughout the years are a testament to the impact of a lifestyle and physical activity tailored to one's needs and environment.

So, what's his secret? Well, he mostly eats traditional food – none of that baguette and sweet spread for breakfast like we used to think was cool. His morning routine is pretty unique – he eats leftovers from dinner, and guess what? It keeps him super energized until dinner.

We used to tease him because we thought real breakfast meant fancy stuff like omelets and ham. But it turns out he was onto something good. He's not a snacker, and he enjoys a drink now and then but never goes overboard. I've never even seen him drunk! He is still enjoying football, walking, and some martial arts.

Now, let's find out how our body's defense system kicks in with the magic of traditional carbs, fats, proteins, and all those fabulous vitamins and minerals.

1.1. Tropical Traditional food activates our body's five defense mechanisms.

Food can "starve our disease and feed our health,"

Dr William Lee

Just like a country uses its military and police forces to defend itself from various threats, our body has five key defense systems: blood vessel formation, regeneration, DNA protection, the immune system, and gut health. Eating traditional foods helps activate these defenses, protecting our body from internal and external threats. Thanks to Dr. William Lee who helped spread this information in his book "Eat to Beat Disease."

The first defense is how our blood vessels form (Angiogenesis). When we eat or breathe, our blood vessels deliver oxygen and nutrients to every cell. Having too many blood vessels can feed diseases like cancer, heart disease, and inflammation, while too few can harm our cells. Luckily, our body knows how to keep the right amount. Just provide it with the right food, and it will take care of the rest.

The second defense is stem cells, which maintain, repair, and regenerate our cells. We can get stem cells through fasting, physical activity, and specific food.

The third defense is our DNA or genes. Certain foods have the power to switch harmful or helpful genes on or off. It just goes to show how important our food choices are for looking after our genes.

The fourth key player is our immune system, and the fifth is our gut, which holds a whopping 70%-80% of our immune defenses. A huge responsibility! Our gut acts as a gatekeeper for our health. Think of it as a battleground filled with different kinds of bacteria. Some bacteria are beneficial and help strengthen our immune system, while others can be harmful and weaken it. We want the good bacteria to dominate so that our gut can thrive. The food we eat can either feed the harmful bacteria, dampening our immune functions or nourish and multiply the beneficial bacteria, boosting our body's defense system.

So basically, eating lots of processed foods, added sugars, dealing with chronic stress, and being around harmful chemicals mess up our body's defenses. But on the bright side, there's a list of specific foods, backed by clinical and scientific research, that support each of the body's five defense systems. These foods are mostly traditional ones. They can either be fermented to make their nutrients more available and easier to digest or cooked fresh from the farm. They include plant-based foods like whole grains, spices, root vegetables, fruits, veggies, legumes, cold-pressed oils, nuts, and seeds. Animal foods like fish, chicken, seafood, and fermented foods are also on the list. Drinks like tea, coffee, and chamomile are included, too. Many of these foods are part of the traditional diets in tropical countries. So, we've got everything we need right at home to boost our body's defenses!

1.2. Traditional foods heal and protect against diseases

Traditional foods in tropical countries share a lot of similarities. When I stroll through a market in Fiji, it feels like I could be in West or Central Africa. I see almost the same kinds of foods I'd find in Uganda, Kenya, Cameroon, Nigeria, or Senegal. Even a variety of yam that I thought was unique to my village turned out to be a Fijian delicacy, too! I've also noticed how similar the dishes in West Africa can be to those in the Caribbean or the Pacific. For example, the way those people from three different continents wrap food in leaves and steam it, or how they use firewood, is just the same.

Let's discover the remarkable healing powers of the key components of traditional food. I'll unravel the secrets of carbohydrates, fat, and protein.

1.2.1.Carbohydrates as the main staple

Consider carbs as your body's ultimate energy boost! Carbs supply the body's fuel in glucose, serving as the go-to source that quickly transforms into the power every cell needs to keep things running smoothly.

The main carbs categories are starches, fibers, and sugars.

Starches are composed of tubers, including cassava roots, yams, cocoyams, sweet potatoes, and taro. Grains are also starchy, and they consist of millet, sorghum, teff, corn, fonio, etc. These foods slowly release glucose in the body.

Fibers are present in traditional plant-based foods such as starches, nuts, seeds, beans, fruits, and vegetables. Fiber is essential for slowing down glucose absorption, ensuring a steady and balanced release of energy. In simple terms, it protects you from experiencing energy crashes. Further details on the types of fibers, including soluble and insoluble fibers, along with their specific roles and health benefits, can be found in Table 4: Carbs & Health Snapshot, in the annex.

Sugars naturally occur in fruits and milk. They zip through digestion, unleashing rapid bursts of glucose for an instant energy kick in the body. This occurs more with fruit juice and less with whole fruits. The presence of fibers in entire fruits slows down the absorption process.

Carbs are also like a treasure trove full of phytochemicals, a fancy term for antioxidants created by plants. These phytochemicals fight off bad stuff in our bodies. Carbs, fibers, and antioxidants work together to help prevent Type 2 diabetes, obesity, certain cancers, and heart disease. So, when you eat carbs, you're not just filling your belly; you're bringing in a team of health superheroes!

Table 4 in the annex lists all carbohydrate types and their role and effect on health.

Tubers and grains

Carbs are a big deal in tropical countries. In my culture, we start enjoying carbs from a very young age. I remember back home, adults would carefully chew cooked cocoyam or plantains and feed the mushy food to babies during meals. It was like a special family time and a way to introduce babies to traditional food early on.

What's cool about tubers and grains is that they have a lot of fiber, which makes us feel full for a long time. They provide a consistent energy flow that lasts all day, keeping us energized. Plus, the fiber in these carbs helps our gut grow friendly bacteria, which team up with other defense systems in our body to keep us strong and healthy.

Tubers and grains have a wide range of antioxidants. They can even be fermented to give our gut some friendly bacteria—probiotics. They're found in many African local staple foods. Take teff, for example. It's a super nutritious grain staple in Ethiopia and Eritrea. People use it to make *Injera*, which is a fermented flatbread-like food. *Injera* gives us the goodness of carbs mentioned above and increases the number of friendly bacteria in the gut. *Injera* has a tangy taste that goes perfectly with spiced meat, lentils, and veggies served with it. It's not just tasty; it helps lower cholesterol, boosts our immune system, and protects us from pesky microbes.

Tubers like cassava are typically peeled before cooking, whereas grains like corn, teff, fonio and millet are ready to cook once you remove the grains. You can prepare tubers and grains by soaking, fermenting, powdering, or combining these methods before cooking. For instance, in East Africa, staples like *Ugali* and *Posho;* in Southern Africa, dishes like *Nshima*; and in West and Central Africa, foods such as *Fufu, Water Fufu*, and *Placali* have a doughy, mashed potato-like consistency. They are made from powdered maize and fermented cassava. These dishes can be paired with various sauces like stews, vegetable-based dishes, and peanut or pumpkin seed sauces.

One unique dish I experienced, introduced by a friend from Sierra Leone, is *Lafidi*. It consists of steamed fonio, raw palm oil, and fermented locust bean powder, also known as *Soumbala* or *Netetou* in West Africa. As you eat, you mix the oil and *Netetou* in fonio, creating a delicious combination. In the Caribbean, they make cassava bread by taking the water out of fresh cassava and baking the mashed cassava. They boil the gathered cassava juice until it becomes brown, creating a delicious syrup known as *Pepperpot*. No need to add sugar to the syrup—cassava juice is naturally sweet enough to satisfy those with a sweet tooth. People in the Caribbean enjoy this Guyanese-Amerindian thick syrup with foods like bread, rice, and steak. These tasty foods contribute to lowering the risk of major chronic diseases.

In the Pacific, the types of readily available carbs can vary from one country to another. In Tonga, sweet potatoes and yams are widely enjoyed, while in Papua New Guinea, sweet potatoes, known as *Kaukau*, along with taro and cassava, are commonly consumed. Different from Africa, grains like maize or millet are less common in the traditional dishes of these Pacific Islands and Caribbean countries. Instead, they enjoy tubers like cassava, sweet potatoes, and yams.

These tubers and grains come straight from the farm, with little processing. They won't cause a spike in our insulin because they give our body the nutrients it loves and understands. They won't just sit in our stomachs, giving us a protruding belly. Instead, they'll spread throughout our body in a beautiful way, feeding each cell with the right amount of glucose and other nutrients.

Having said that, with gluten-related health issues like sensitivity, intolerance, and celiac disease becoming more prevalent, many people are now searching for gluten-free alternatives. And where better to find them than in the tropical food world? Up next, I'll dive into why cassava flour is not only tastier but also a healthier option than wheat for our baked treats. The best part is it not only meets dietary needs but also retains a delicious taste! Plus, the availability of cassava flour all year round in tropical countries makes it a convenient and accessible option.

The Tropical Story of Wheat: From Beginning to Now

Did you know that the wheat we have today is different from what it was before the twentieth century? Over time, through various crossings, the height of wheat plants has been reduced by about 10 cm. This change was made to make Western countries more self-sufficient in wheat production, as it is a staple food, especially after World War II when food was scarce. Wheat serves as the basis for pasta, pastries, and many baked goods in Western countries.

Wheat became popular in tropical countries much later, changing food preferences and creating a demand for easy-to-get and cooked foods. We've adapted to using highly processed wheat flour to make desserts, snacks like *Puff Puffs, Haitian Patty*, Trinidad and Tobago *Double* which is a sandwich of two fried flatbreads filled with curried chickpeas.

The heavy dependence of tropical countries on wheat became glaringly evident when Ukraine and Russia, major wheat suppliers, got deeply involved in conflict with each other. As they focused on the war, wheat supply was drying up in Tropical countries, posing

a real threat to food availability and affordability. Meanwhile, traditional root crops are abundantly available locally. It might be time for our traditional staples to reclaim the spotlight that wheat has taken. Perhaps it's a call to go back to the locally available foods.

From Wheat to Gluten-Free Tubers and Grains: A Growing Trend

In the Western world, an increasing number of people are trying different tropical foods because of gluten-related health issues. They're experimenting with alternatives like maize, cassava, and millet pasta instead of wheat. Nut-based flours are also catching on. The West is slowly changing its eating habits to tackle the challenges of wheat, possibly worsened by genetic modifications.

On the flip side, tropical regions present a puzzle. While the West is frantically searching for gluten-free options, these tropical areas, already rich in naturally gluten-free foods, are finding new ways to use imported and highly processed wheat flour. Understanding the missing link in this pattern is a bit tricky.

Now, if you're on the hunt for a gluten-free option that's really close to wheat, cassava flour is the way to go. It's similar to wheat flour in texture, with a mild taste compared to other gluten-free options. You can use it in recipes like cakes, bread, cookies, crackers, and even banana bread. The key is to measure it by weight instead of volume and adjust the water accordingly. And here's the fun part — you can mix it with other gluten-free flours like teff, maize, or millet to add creativity and change up the taste. It's like becoming a gluten-free baking wizard! Let's dive into this "exotic" cassava alternative and see what it has to offer!

Why Choose Gluten-Free Cassava Flour Over Wheat Flour?

Cassava crops are the main income source for millions of farmers across tropical countries. Choosing cassava flour supports local farmers, makes our community healthier, and boosts the economy of tropical regions.

Now, let me give you two reasons why picking cassava flour over wheat flour improves your health.

Comparison 1: Processing Methods of Wheat and Cassava

When it comes to cassava, our ancestors were pretty smart—they knew it contained natural toxins like cyanide. They figured out ways to get rid of it using traditional methods like soaking, fermenting, squeezing out the water, and boiling. The cool thing is, these tricks get rid of a lot of cyanide, like 80- 95%! When we boil cassava, around 90% of that cyanide disappears in 15 minutes. Soaking and fermenting cassava helps us kick out even more cyanide while making it easier to digest and more nutritious. These methods bring the cyanide to safer levels, as recommended by the World Health Organization.

Cyanide naturally occurs in varying amounts in some fruits and nuts, so it's nothing new in the food world. As long as we keep it at safe levels, we can avoid health issues like thyroid problems and brain disorders.

On the other hand, when wheat goes through the milling process, the bran—the nutritious outer layer—gets removed. This strips the flour of essential nutrients and fiber, turning it into empty calories. As a result, it becomes tougher to digest compared to whole wheat, which is already challenging for our gut.

Comparison 2: Wheat vs Cassava - Effects on Gut Health

Gluten-containing foods such as wheat can pose a serious challenge to our gut.

Imagine our gut is a busy town with lots of helpers known as friendly bacteria and a protective barrier. Like any processed food, gluten can be a troublemaker in this town. It can upset the helpers and damage the protective barrier, like when a good team isn't working well together.

Now, here's the important part: our gut town is like the boss of our immune system, hosting about 70-80% of it. It is like a superhero squad defending our bodies. If our gut town is happy and has lots of different friendly bacteria, our superhero squad is strong and ready to protect us!

When we eat foods that aren't good for our gut, we lose the friendly bacteria and let the bad ones take over. This condition is called dysbiosis. It doesn't just mess with our gut; it also affects our brain, showing how gut bacteria can influence more than just our digestion. Dysbiosis gradually makes the protective filter barriers in our gut and brain leaky. This is known as "leaky gut" when it affects our gut and "leaky brain" when it affects our brain.

Our brain's filter is called the blood-brain barrier, and it keeps harmful stuff out, similar to how you'd pick out bones when eating fish to avoid choking. If this barrier becomes too leaky, it can let in harmful things, potentially leading to problems like Alzheimer's.

A leaky gut can also allow bad stuff to enter our bloodstream, leading to inflammation, bloating, stomach cramps, and gluten intolerance. But it doesn't stop there; it can also lead to bigger problems like obesity, heart disease, diabetes, and brain diseases.

Caring for our gut is like protecting our brain and the rest of our body. If our gut goes wrong, it's like opening the door to anything and everything. That's why it is crucial to provide prebiotics, which is food our friendly bacteria need to keep our gut healthy. Cassava appears as the perfect food which contains powerful prebiotic. Other foods such as beans, lentils, veggies and fruits also have prebiotics.

Besides feeding our friendly bacteria, we also need to diversify them. Different types of friendly bacteria give us better protection, just like you need shoes for your feet, sunglasses for your eyes, and clothes for your body. You can't use one for the other. Each type of friendly bacteria, called probiotic likes different foods. We can find them in fermented foods from milk, grains, and tubers like cassava. Check the section "Traditional Food Preservation Techniques Boost our Immune System" below for more information on fermentation.

Choosing traditional foods that are naturally gluten-free, like cassava, is a win for our gut health. It keeps our immune system in top shape, while wheat and other gluten-containing foods may threaten our body's defense system.

"Prevention is not just better than cure, prevention is the cure"

Pr. Robert Lustig

Vegetables and fruits

Let's explore the vibrant tropical world, where a variety of delicious fruits and veggies captivate our senses. Join me on a journey through tropical countries, where leafy green vegetables often steal the show as the meal's star. In the Pacific and Caribbean paradises, a splash of coconut milk turns veggies into culinary masterpieces. Meanwhile, across Africa, it's a symphony of sautéed veggies in red palm oil, seasoned with the savory notes of dry fish or crayfish. But In Africa, the magic unfolds when greens are combined with saucy creations, with or without nuts, resulting in a meal that is not only delicious but also a rich source of natural plant antioxidants known as polyphenols. It's a culinary experience that combines flavor and health benefits in one.

Now, let's talk polyphenols – the unsung antioxidant heroes found in fruits, veggies, nuts, seeds, and beyond. Our bodies crave a variety of these antioxidants, and the color and flavor of fruits or veggies are the secret code revealing the types of polyphenols within. So, here's the secret to unlocking a treasure trove of antioxidants: savoring a mix of local fruits and veggies.

Enter the superheroes of the vegetable world – leafy greens packed with polyphenols, acting like a battalion for our health. Veggies like cassava leaves, watercress, cocoyam, and taro leaves aren't just nutritious; they outshine foreign greens like spinach. Amaranth leaves, whether known as "*folon*" in Cameroon, *Dodo leaves* in Uganda, or *Tubua/Bhaji* in Fiji, carry their own antioxidant power. Make dishes like *Nzap lah*[3] and *Eru*[4] in Cameroon, *Fumbwa*[5] in Congo, *Palusami*[6] in Fiji, or mixed veggies in Nigeria a regular part of your weekly menu, and you've just struck health gold. It's like boosting your bones, building a fortress against diseases like cancer and diabetes, and ensuring your brain stays in tip-top shape. Leafy greens are a protective shield for our body, and they taste pretty darn good too!

And don't forget about moringa trees, which offer delicious and nutritious leaves, seeds, and pods! You can enjoy moringa in so many ways. People in the Caribbean and African countries enjoy these leaves in similar ways. They boil or lightly roast the seeds, cook the fresh leaves in sauces, dips, stews, or blend them in smoothies and sprinkle them on salads. The only difference is the ingredients used. You can also make tea from the dried leaves. Drying moringa even improves its shelf life without losing its nutritional value.

Known as "Mother's best friend" or the "miracle tree," the moringa tree thrives in dry climates and truly lives up to its name. Moringa is a complete protein, making it an excellent substitute for eggs, meat, or fish. It has 7 times more vitamin C than oranges, 10 times more vitamin A than carrots, 17 times more calcium than milk, 9 times more protein than yogurt, 15 times more potassium than bananas, and 25 times more iron than spinach. The leaves are

---

[3] *Nzap Lah* is the Jieumba term (a dialect of the Dshang-Cameroon language) used to refer to a traditional dish of stir-fried huckleberry leaves commonly enjoyed in western Cameroon.

[4] *Eru* or *Afang* is a traditional delicacy from Cameroon and Nigeria. It features Eru leaves a wild type of spinach (also referred to as "Ukazi" in Nigeria), known for their robust texture, alongside a unique spinach variety called "waterleaf". Combined with palm oil, crayfish, smoked fish, meat, and cow skin, it offers a rich and flavorful dish. Typically enjoyed with a side of water fufu or gari, both of which are dough-like pastes made from fermented cassava.

[5] *Fumbwa* is a comforting Congolese dish crafted from Eru/Ukazi leafy greens, simmered with red palm oil and ground roasted peanuts to produce a rich and creamy stew.

[6] *Palusami*, a cherished traditional Pacific Island dish, comprises bundles of taro leaves enveloping a filling of coconut milk and onion. Variations may include chicken, and fish, with ingredient preferences differing across countries. For example, in Fiji, the addition of tomato, garlic, and corned beef is favored. Taro leaves can be either steamed, mashed and mixed with the ingredients or used to wrap them before steaming, or cooking in an earth oven. Palusami pairs well with taro, cassava, or other tubers.

especially good for treating malnutrition in children—countries like Senegal and Benin have been using it for that purpose. The leaves also help increase breastmilk production in nursing moms. Want to make sure your baby doesn't run out of milk? Moringa could be the answer! Just 6 spoonfuls of leaf powder can meet a woman's daily iron and calcium needs during pregnancy. Moringa is fantastic for lowering high blood pressure. It also packs a punch with its anti-inflammatory, anticancer, antidiabetic, antiulcer, and antimicrobial properties. It's like having a natural medicine cabinet in a plant!

Just be careful though—consuming more than 70 grams of moringa a day can lead to too much iron in your body, causing gut issues and other health problems.

Feeling a bit worn out and in need of a pick-me-up? Well, tropical countries have the perfect solution – nature's very own energy drink in the form of sugar cane sticks. Just give them a good suck! Another fantastic option is coconut water, especially from those vibrant green coconuts. Personally, they're my top pick because they're incredibly fresh and sweet. I go for the ones with thicker flesh, so I can scoop it up with a spoon and savor it for longer.

There's also this delicious energy-dense snack called *Mounou Mounouk* from Northern Chad. It's a brownish paste made from pounded dried dates, lightly cooked over low heat with groundnut oil, and seasoned with nigella seeds. It's mainly enjoyed with tea. *Mounou Mounouk* is not only tasty and naturally sweet but also packed with energy—no need to buy energy bars! This naturally energizing option has no added sugar. Nature did its magic by packing these treats with sugar, fibers, and fat, creating a delightful and natural way to boost our energy levels!

Budget-Friendly Guide for Starchy Foods, Veggies, and Fruits:

➔ Choose fresh and locally grown tubers, grains, fruits and veggies for the best health benefits. Local foods are better because they have yet to travel long distances, losing their antioxidant power. They're packed with more nutrients. Eat them as fresh as you can. If fresh isn't an option, go for the frozen version—it's the next best thing!

➔ When you live in western countries, farmers market are a place you can find fresh and organic produce from local farmers. They are more nutritious and tasty. Whole Foods Market is also a good option for those living in North America. But if you're aiming for budget-friendly and nutritious choices, frozen veggies is the way to go!

➔ Eat greens at least two to three times a week to reap maximum health benefits.

➔ When you cook greens, don't boil them and toss the water! You're getting rid of vitamins and minerals. Some love doing this when making sautéed Folon, Njama Njama, or other greens. Sautéing them directly not only gives you the best flavor and taste but also keeps all the good nutrients in the greens. So, skip the boiling and enjoy the full benefits of your tasty greens!

➜ Don't cook your veggies for too long, or you'll lose a lot of the good stuff in them. Try simmering them at low heat instead – that way, they will remain crunchy and keep most of the nutrients!

1.2.2. Fats (Tropical oils and more)

Who can resist the allure of delicious food, right? And let's be honest – fat is the secret that makes everything taste amazing. Picture this: dipping roasted plantain in raw red palm oil or drizzling coconut cream on veggies – pure yum! In tropical countries, folks have mastered the art of using various fats, from oils and fish to meat, insects, nuts, and seeds.

But here's the plot twist – fat hasn't always had a fair reputation. Maybe it's because fat brings a whopping 9 calories per gram, more than protein (4 calories/g) and carbs (4 calories/g) combined. Some misconceptions have led people to believe that indulging in fat will make them gain weight, scaring them away from its delights. But let me drop some truth bombs – try binging on sugary treats like ice cream, cakes, cookies, pizza, and dessert for a week, and not only will you gain weight, but you'll also feel miserable and tired. Now, flip the script and immerse yourself in a week of high-fat delights like *Mbongo tchobi*[7], *Nnam owondo*[8], and *Kokoda*[9]. Don't stop there—try some *Liboke* or *Luwombo* (meat or fish steamed in banana leaves), too, all while sticking to a low-carb diet. Brace yourself because this journey could lead to shedding those extra pounds and surfing the energy wave like a true champion.

Why? Because fat is packed with concentrated energy. It doesn't just make food taste better; it gives a long-lasting energy boost without crashes. Plus, a low-carb, high-fat diet gradually uses up glucose stores, leaving them insufficient to fuel the whole body. This triggers fat cells to open up, and release energy, leading to weight loss. Plus, fat plays a crucial role in our body's stash of fat-friendly antioxidants like A, D, E, and K (especially K2). These antioxidants are most plentiful and better absorbed when eaten with fat. And here's the kicker – our traditional foods are a goldmine of these wonders. Steering clear of fat in our diet could be a health gamble,

---

[7] Mbongo Tchobi (Cameroonian): A delectable sauce ranging from light to dark brown, crafted with fish, special spices, and red palm oil. Cook it directly in the pot or steam it in banana leaves for an authentic touch. Best enjoyed with tubers.

[8] Nnam Owondo (Cameroonian): Dive into the richness of roasted peanuts paste, seasoned with crayfish and spices. Whether cooked in a pot or steamed in banana leaves, it pairs perfectly with tubers for a satisfying meal.

[9] Kokoda (Pacific countries): Experience Fiji's national dish featuring just-caught diced fish marinated in lime juice. Complemented by coconut milk and diced veggies, it's a refreshing and flavorful delight. Kokoda is largely enjoyed in the Pacific countries.

as we might end up deficient in these key antioxidants. And trust me, these vitamins and antioxidants? They're the superheroes defending us from diseases and the aging game. Take vitamin A, for example – its retinol is used in cosmetics to battle wrinkles. Now, picture what vitamin A could do for our organs when we get it from our meals! It's time to make friends with Fat and rethink our partnership. It's an ally, not an enemy. Let's celebrate the good fats – the flavorful and health-boosting kind!

Cooking Oils

Ever strolled down the grocery store aisles and felt like you've entered a haven for oil enthusiasts? Shelves lined with oils flaunting fancy labels, each in a fierce competition to be crowned the ultimate champion. Some boldly shout "cholesterol-free" or "trans-fat-free," while others boast about their "saturated fat-free" status. It's like a showdown of oil glamour, and each bottle is vying for the coveted title of the best in the game. It's a jungle out there, and the competition is fierce, making the choices seem endless and, frankly, a bit perplexing.

Here's the kicker – the Western world has successfully convinced us that tropical oils are the villains of the oil world, often dismissed due to their high saturation levels. It's like they've thrown shade on Tropical traditional oils, making us fear them. But hold on – I'm here to challenge that belief and spill the beans on why tropical oil should be our first choice. First, let's dissect the common vegetable oil gracing many kitchen shelves. Then, armed with some science facts, we'll embark on a journey into the world of tropical oils. Strap in for the oil exploration ahead!

Refined Vegetable Oil

Let's talk about those oils we often find labeled as "vegetable oil" or "seed oil" – canola, sunflower, safflower, corn oil, cotton oil, and the infamous margarine. They're like the popular kids in the oil world, but here's the catch – they've been getting a bit too much hype! These oils come with a hefty dose of omega-6 fats, and let me tell you, in high amounts, they can be downright inflammatory. And guess where else omega-6 is throwing a party? Yup, in nearly all processed foods and sauces. Now, when you don't have enough omega-3 to keep the balance, things can take a nosedive into health trouble territory.

Here's the ideal scenario – the omega-3 to omega-6 ratio should be a sweet 1:3 (some scientists say 1:2). But brace yourself for reality – it's usually an unbalanced 1:20, and that's a red flag. Why? Because this skewed ratio might spark inflammation, crank up the bad cholesterol, give the boot to the good one, and even pave the way for serious heart issues like atherosclerosis and Coronary Heart Disease.

Now, these vegetable oils flaunt a type of omega-3 called ALA, but there's a catch – our body has to do a little makeover, turning ALA into essential fatty acids so our cells can groove to the right rhythm. The glitch? This transformation isn't always a smooth operator, meaning you might not be getting enough of those vital omega-3 fatty acids from your favorite vegetable oils.

Let's delve into the manufacturing process. When crafting these oils, there's a significant concern about the procedures in place. The oil initially appears brown and isn't very pleasant in terms of smell, so they decide to give it a makeover. It's like when you use chemicals to dye your dull-looking hair and give it a vibrant, pretty color that doesn't change your natural hair's inherent nature. In this case, they're transforming vegetable oil from brown to a sunny yellow. However, it's not just a dab of bleach; additional chemicals, sometimes corrosive like acid or alkali, are added. The entire mixture undergoes a filtering process, and to enhance the chemical transformation, petrochemicals like Hexane are introduced to the mix.

At the end of this chemical symphony, oils like canola, sunflower, cottonseed, safflower, and soybean all come out looking like long-lost siblings—a pretty golden yellow. But that's not all; they've all been through pretty much the same chemical *wahala* (i.e., trouble in West African Pidgin language). That's the not-so-natural truth about those oils we use so often.

Tropical Oils

In many parts of Africa, traditional cooking oils are mainly red palm, groundnut, ghee, coconut, avocado, and sesame oil. The most common ones are palm oil and coconut oil. In some places in East Africa, they didn't use oil traditionally. Instead, they used nuts and the fatty part of animal meat for fat. In the Pacific and the Caribbean traditions, coconut oil is central to the diet. Those oils have kept generations healthy before modernization.

All oils have two types of fats: saturated and unsaturated. Tropical oils like palm oil (50% saturated fat) and coconut oil (90% saturated fat) have more saturated fat. Some people say this saturated fat could cause heart disease.

But let me take you back to a time when heart problems were the talk of the town in the USA. The worry escalated when President Franklin Roosevelt passed away in 1945 due to heart disease linked to untreated high blood pressure. That's when the USA decided to roll up its sleeves and dive into some serious detective work. Pouring a ton of resources into research, they pointed fingers at saturated fat, thinking it was the troublemaker causing heart diseases. The solution? Convince everyone to cut back on it, hoping it would be the magic fix for the heart disease puzzle.

Surprisingly, despite nationwide efforts to reduce saturated fat consumption, heart diseases persisted. It seemed like the villain they were chasing wasn't the real culprit. Enter the

Framingham studies, one of the most robust in the research field, to set the record straight. These studies flipped the script, revealing that saturated fat wasn't causing heart diseases—it was, in fact, a heart-healthy helper, contributing to our overall well-being!

And it's not just Framingham; lots of other studies have high-fived these findings on saturated fat. So, it turns out that enjoying some roasted cocoyam with palm oil or some coconut would make our bodies happy after all!

And speaking of saturated fat, did you know that the first food we had, breast milk, is about 50% saturated fat? This highlights that right from our first days, our body is loudly declaring its need for saturated fat. If this doesn't signal what our bodies require, then what else could it be? Saturated fat plays a key role in our body's cell walls. Interestingly, too little saturated fat in our diet weakens our cell walls, making us more likely to get sick. So, it turns out that what our body craves from the beginning might just be the secret to keeping us strong and healthy!

Now, let's turn our attention to the red palm oil.

Red Palm oil is the "Tropical Olive Oil."

For over 5000 years, African ancestors have been in on the secret of red palm oil, making it a staple in traditional dishes across West and Central Africa. They're not just into the trendy parts – every bit of the palm fruit, from the inside to the seeds, is put to good use because, well, they're bursting with goodness.

Now, meet a relative in the palm oil family – palm kernel oil. It's sleek and black, and we lovingly call it *Nsouhèmenang* in my village. The name combines *Nsouheli*, meaning slip, and *linang*, meaning life. So, *Nsouhèmenang* washes away anything that could threaten our lives. No wonder we've been using it traditionally for medicinal purposes. Our forefathers knew its medicinal benefits. Palm kernel oil is versatile in several West African villages, from skincare to haircare. It's a true multitasker!

On the flip side, the red palm oil from the juicy inside of the fruit takes center stage in the kitchen, adding flavor and a hefty dose of vitamins A and E. Each oil brings its distinct flavor and health advantages to the table.

For now, we will focus on red palm oil and see what distinguishes the refined and unrefined versions.

Refined palm oil

Refined palm oil is like the distant cousin of its naturally red counterpart, and let me tell you, they're not on speaking terms. Why? Because it goes through a bleaching process, stripping away that vibrant red hue and leaving behind a more neutral color and flavor. Now, you might be wondering where this refined player hangs out – well, it's a VIP in the worlds of soaps, detergents, cosmetics, and even the food industries.

You'll spot it playing a crucial role in the making of chocolates, biscuits, crackers, and other baked goodies. Not only does it do wonders for enhancing flavor, but it also extends the shelf life of these tempting treats. And guess who else is a fan? The fast food industry, where refined palm oil takes the spotlight for frying up mass-produced delights. It comes with a damaging effect on our health. It's the culprit often used to tarnish the reputation of its naturally vibrant cousin, red palm oil.

Unrefined red palm oil

For ages, our ancestors in Africa have been cooking up something special in their kitchens—a magical elixir known as red palm oil. It is a rich, reddish hue with an earthy taste that adds extra oomph to our favorite dishes. It's the secret ingredient our grandmother swears by, and for good reason.

This treasure comes straight from the heart of the palm fruit, packed with goodness like beta-carotene and a squad of antioxidants. It's the culinary maestro behind dishes like *Coki*, *Moyi Moyi* or *Olele*, where cowpea paste is mixed with red palm oil, spices (optional), taro leaves and steamed in banana leaves. There's also *Mbongo Tchobi*, a spicy dark brown dish made with meat or fish in palm oil. The list goes on to include Fumbwa, *Pundu*[10], *Topsi banana*[11], *Sauce graine*[12], okra sauce, and the mighty *Egusi sauce*[13]. So, the next time you're savoring those mouthwatering West and Central African flavors, know that red palm oil is the unsung hero making it all happen.

Now, let's delve into how scientific advancements have not only lifted palm oil from its negative reputation but also unraveled the truth to set the record straight.

---

[10] Pundu is a Congolese and Central African dish. It consist of pounded cassava leaves cooked with red palm oil, garlic , smoked fish, green onion, and various spices.

[11] Topsi banana is a delicious dish from Cameroon featuring groundnut paste, red palm oil, and unripe bananas as its main ingredients.

[12] Sauce graine is a delectable West African dish, highly favored in Côte d'Ivoire. It's crafted from palm nut pulp, from which a creamy sauce is extracted and cooked with a mixture of seafood and meat. This delightful meal is typically enjoyed with pounded banana or yam.

[13] Egusi sauce is a flavorful sauce from Central-West Africa, prepared with pumpkin seeds, red palm oil, greens, and a blend of spices. Okra can be added to bring some slimy texture.

The resurgence of red Palm oil

In the realm of recent discussions, palm oil has found itself under a cloud of criticism, especially when the spotlight falls on its refined version rather than the unrefined alternative. Like many oils, refined palm oil might not be the health hero we'd hope for. Its production can give birth to some not-so-friendly chemicals that have been associated with inflammation and various diseases, even the ominous cancer tag. Unsurprisingly, this questionable oil frequently finds its way into the realms of processed and fast foods, adding a layer of concern to its already dubious reputation.

Beyond health matters, ethical alarms echo about the broader impacts of palm oil production on our environment, wildlife, and communities. These concerns echo similar issues faced by other large plantations and farms, painting palm oil plantations with a similar brush. What adds a unique twist to this tale is the surprising fact that India (17%) and China (17%) top the charts as global producers despite not being heavy consumers domestically. In contrast, Africa (11%) produces less but seems to have a stronger love affair with palm oil. And in a twist of fate, even with global criticisms, Malaysia and Indonesia are embracing palm oil in their cooking, aligning their culinary practices with those of Central and West Africans.

Discovering the wonders of red palm oil is like stumbling upon a hidden treasure in the world of healthy choices. Back in 2016, a savvy researcher named Lucci P. and his team from the University of Udine in Italy hailed red palm oil as "The tropical equivalent of Olive oil." Now, that's a statement that could shake things up. Notably, numerous other researchers have independently reached similar conclusions. The spotlight on red palm oil has intensified, drawing more research attention that resounds with the same compelling results.

Interestingly, the groundbreaking studies showcasing red palm oil's awesomeness often stay low-key, not stealing the limelight. Imagine if everyone knew that red palm oil is as fantastic for our health as the beloved olive oil. Mind-blowing, right?

This revelation could be a game-changer, challenging the negative vibe surrounding palm oil. If we all hopped on the red palm oil train, it could not only boost our health but also show some love to local producers.

The more we embrace red palm oil, the less room there is for other not-so-healthy oils like vegetable oils. And guess who's not thrilled about that? Big food companies with pockets as deep as Lake Tanganyika. They stand to lose millions, and let's be real, they won't let go without a fight.

But our secret weapon is knowledge. Armed with the truth about red palm oil, we can flip the script on this narrative. It's as simple as choosing the healthiest option for ourselves. In this battle of oils, we hold the power to make the better, tastier, and healthier choice. Let's change the game, one drop of red palm oil at a time!

Health benefits of red palm oil

Now, here are the science-based reasons why we need to make red palm oil our ally and not our enemy!

Boosts Immune System: Red palm oil contains particular nutrients and antioxidants, like vitamin E and Betacarotene, which turn into Vitamin A, helping keep our immune system strong and age slower.

Supports Brain Health: Red palm oil antioxidants can make our brains work better, making us smarter. Plus, it helps guard against diseases like Alzheimer's.

Fights Cancer: Red palm oil lowers the risk of certain cancers and can even improve chemotherapy's adverse effects.

Keeps Eyes Healthy: It protects our eyes from problems like cataracts and other diseases that can worsen our eyesight.

Heart Protection: Just like extra virgin olive oil, red palm oil protects our hearts in many ways:

- O It prevents artery Problems by lowering the chance of artery issues like thrombosis and atherosclerosis.
- O It lowers the bad cholesterol (LDL) and boosts the good cholesterol (HDL)
- O It controls blood pressure by keeping it in check and protecting us from hypertension.

Fights Inflammation and Diseases: Red palm oil helps reduce our body's production of something harmful called "free radicals." Free radicals are unstable and troublesome molecules that need to latch onto something to survive. They usually go after fats, proteins, and DNA. When they attach to these, they mess up how our body processes fats and proteins, causing inflammation, DNA damage, and early aging. They're a big cause of chronic diseases like heart disease, cataracts, cancer, Type 2 diabetes, and inflammatory conditions.

Interestingly, our body naturally produces free radicals as part of its normal processes, so we can't really avoid them. However, we can control the free radicals from external sources like X-rays, cigarette smoke, processed foods, car exhaust, and other pollutants.

Thankfully, we can fight free radicals and cut down their production by consuming natural antioxidants found in nutritious traditional foods like palm oil.

As evident, even though red palm oil has more saturated fat than olive oil (see Table 2 below), it has still shown heart-healthy benefits similar to extra virgin olive oil.

Table 2: Comparison of fat Content in olive oil and red palm oil

Oil types	Saturated fat	Monounsaturated fat (omega-9)	Polyunsaturated fat (Omega 3 et 6)
Extra virgin Olive oil	10%	73%	11%
Unrefined Red palm oil	50%	40%	10%
Fat Comparison	Higher in palm oil	Higher in olive oil	Almost the same

Note: The fat composition in each oil can vary slightly depending on the quality of the olives and palm fruits used.

Coconut Oil

Now, imagine a world where coconuts reign supreme – well, that's the reality in the Caribbean, Pacific islands, and Africa. These places have been coconut enthusiasts for ages, making the humble coconut a superstar in their kitchens and beauty routines.

Stroll through the Caribbean, Fiji, or the Pacific, and you'll see coconuts everywhere. It's not just a fruit; it's a lifestyle! People work culinary magic, whipping up homemade coconut milk and cream from scratch to add that extra oomph to their dishes. And here's the fun part: no worries if you're not in the mood to grate your coconut! Just swing by your local market or supermarket, and they'll take care of the grating for you—leaving you with the delight of squeezing out fresh coconut milk.

In Fijian communities, coconut grating has become a friendly competition. Yes, you heard it right—they gather at events to see who can grate coconuts at lightning speed. Talk about turning a chore into a party!

Travel to Africa, and while coconut fever might not be as widespread, coastal areas with coconut trees are in on the action. They use coconuts in the same cool ways—cooking, beauty rituals, you name it. And when they whip up coconut oil the traditional way, it's all about keeping it unrefined—a true celebration of coconut goodness.

So, whether you're savoring a coconut-infused dish in the Pacific or witnessing a coconut grating showdown in Fiji, one thing's for sure – coconuts are the real MVPs, bringing joy and flavor to communities across the globe.

Virgin coconut oil is a powerhouse containing about 90% saturated fats and 9% unsaturated fats. However, there's something special in the coconut oil called lauric acid, which makes up a whopping 50% of the fat content.

Lauric acid is like magic fuel for our body. It's a special kind of fat that the body quickly turns into energy without going through complex processes. It's used in the body to make energy directly. This means it can boost our energy almost as quickly as whole tubers and grains! Lauric acid is not only found in coconut oil but is also used in things like infant formulas, drinks for athletes, and Intravenous infusions.

Lauric acid, combined with the antioxidants in coconuts, becomes our heart's loyal protector. It's like a shield, ready to fend off chronic diseases and may even tackle cancer.

Just like unrefined palm oil, virgin coconut oil can swoop in and be our defense against heart disease, type 2 diabetes, and, yes, the notorious cancer. Some studies even throw in a bonus: coconut oil might be a secret weapon against infectious diseases. Talk about a multi-talented sidekick!

So, the next time you reach for that virgin coconut oil, know that you're not just adding flavor to your dishes—you're inviting a health ally to the party!

Groundnut oil or Peanut Oil

Take a journey back to the vibrant kitchens of 1980s Cameroon, where my mom, the epitome of beauty, love, and elegance, ruled with an array of flavors. Peanut oil danced alongside the ever-present palm oil.

In addition to being a full-time teacher and mere culinary virtuoso, my mom was a true Wonder Woman with remarkable organizational skills. She had a high standard in the kitchen and would not settle for less. She embraced new recipes with zest, dedicating weekends to preparing batches of meals with groundnut and red palm oils for the upcoming week. She'd then store these delicious creations in the freezer. This made our lives easy – all we had to do was warm them up or boil some tubers and grains to go with the ready-made sauces. Thanks to her passion and efficiency, our kitchen felt like a harmonious masterpiece.

Now, let's fast-forward a bit. A culinary change happened, and like magic, groundnut oil gracefully moved aside, letting vegetable oil steal the spotlight. Groundnut oil was deeply rooted in African culture, and even now, the vegetable oil that took its place hasn't quite wiped away the memories of this cultural favorite. So much so that in Cameroon and some African countries, folks still casually call any vegetable oil "groundnut oil." Ah, the stories these kitchens hold!

To avoid a culinary identity crisis, it's crucial to play detective and ask the right questions. When someone mentions "groundnut oil," it's better to clarify which type—is it sunflower, cotton, corn, or the generic vegetable oil blend?

I became curious about why groundnut oil disappeared from African kitchens, so I set out on a journey to learn more about the whole story. As I delved into the mystery, I unearthed a revelation—it wasn't a mere culinary trend; deeper forces were at play.

Allergic reactions to peanuts made groundnut oil slowly fall out of favor. Interestingly, while about 2% of the Western population is allergic to peanuts, in tropical countries, such allergies are rare. This means for the majority of people, a significant 98%, peanuts aren't a problem. So, why did the small percentage of peanut allergies lead to avoiding groundnut oil? And why aren't shrimp, which can also trigger severe allergic reactions, treated the same way? It makes me question the real reason behind groundnut oil's decline. Further digging revealed concerns about the health risks of improperly handling groundnuts. But food mishandling risks aren't unique to peanuts; they apply to all foods. Plus, we have government food regulations ensuring safe handling, so where did groundnut oil go?

Unrefined groundnut oil is rich in nutrients like protein and vitamin E. It also has a balanced mix of fats: about 50% omega-9 (monounsaturated fatty acids), 30% omega-3 and omega-6 (polyunsaturated fatty acids), and 14% saturated fatty acids. Sounds technical, but it's basically a heart-friendly combo that our ticker will thank us for. In the oil world, unrefined groundnut oil proudly shares similarities with the revered extra virgin olive oil. Like olive and palm oils, it does a great job at lowering bad cholesterol and tricky triglycerides, keeping our hearts happy and healthy.

In the world of oils, unrefined groundnut oil stands tall with a significant amount of the same type of fat as the revered olive oil. Unrefined groundnut oil, like olive and palm oils, lowers bad cholesterol (LDL) and troublesome triglycerides, reducing the chances of heart disease.

The Tropical Oils In Summary

Just like extra virgin olive oil, unrefined tropical oils are full of healthy fats and antioxidants that fight diseases. Even though I didn't dive too deep into avocado oil, it's quite similar to olive oil in terms of fat content. They both are rich in omega-9. However, unlike extra virgin olive oil, extra virgin avocado oil is great for cooking at higher temperatures. Tropical oils options abound!

So, what's the geography lesson? Peanuts, palm nuts, avocados, and coconuts thrive in tropical lands, while olives claim their cozy spots in countries like Spain, Italy, and Greece—that's Europe and the Western world! They've got a grip on information and are savvy enough to avoid shooting themselves in the foot.

It's over to us, the incredible individuals from Africa, the Caribbean, the Pacific, Asia, and all the fellow Tropical oil enthusiasts. Let's take the lead and champion the goodness of Tropical oils, letting their goodness shine. After all, they've got the health benefits, and now they've got the squad to sing their praises.

Maybe it's high time we hit the rewind button on our oil choices and go back to the classics our ancestors swore by for centuries. Sure, they didn't have fancy Western degrees, but they were practically scientists in their own right. They knew the secrets of these oils without needing a modern school to teach them.

But hey, just because tropical oils are good for us doesn't mean we should go crazy pouring them into the food we eat. Like any healthy oil, they've got their dos and don'ts. So, consider this your go-to manual for tropical oils, with some key rules to follow for maximum benefits.

Manual for tropical oils:

Choose the Right Kind of oil

Always pick the organic and cold pressed version of your tropical oil for the best health benefits. Reddish with an earthy flavor for red palm oil, colorless with a strong fresh scent for coconut oil, and light golden with a mild peanut flavor for peanut oil.

Use oil in Moderation

Use oils wisely! Imagine your *Coki* glowing with that vibrant orange-red hue or your *Egusi sauce* with its awesome mix of red and golden pumpkin seed colors. These dishes are a total flavor blast that we adore in West and Central Africa. But don't worry about the amount of oil needed to bring out that taste. Remember, it's all going to be shared, so the oil you're using will be divided among family members. Seriously, oil does make these dishes delicious! Go ahead and add a good splash of red palm oil or another tropical oil to boost the tastiness of your meal. Just make sure not to hog all the *Coki* yourself—spread the love and the food around so everyone gets just the right touch of oiliness.

Cooking Method Matters

Our ancestors used smart cooking methods that were tasty and healthy. These methods included steaming, boiling, baking, cooking using an earth oven, and roasting. Frying is not one of them.

Nuts and Seeds and Other Plant-Based Fat

Ready to boost your immune system and show love to your heart and brain? Well, nuts and seeds are the secret ingredients for that! They're like tiny powerhouses, jam-packed with vitamins, minerals, omega-3, and omega-6. Now, there's a whole variety of these wonders – we're talking African walnut or *Ukpa fruit* in Nigeria, *Likabo Likana* in southern Cameroon, coconuts, chestnuts or *Ivi* in Fiji, *Marula nuts*, bitter kola nuts, pumpkin seeds, sesame seeds, macadamia, almond, cashew nuts, peanuts, and the list goes on. Each one brings unique benefits to the table, so mixing it up and enjoying a variety is a great idea.

Our ancestors were culinary geniuses with these nuts and seeds, whipping delicious meals. They knew how to blend flavors to create dishes that tasted amazing and kept their bodies in tip-top shape. Think of traditional dishes from Tropical places as works of art for our health! And the cool thing is, we can use nuts and seeds in so many ways – boil, roast, grill, grind, or munch on them raw. It's a nutty world out there, and it's time to savor the goodness!

Guess what makes African sauces extra delicious and wonderfully thick? It's the magic touch of nuts and seeds! Let's take a taste tour: there's *Mafe*, a West African wonder made with peanuts, and *Egusi sauce*, a pumpkin seed sensation. Now, head over to Cameroon, and you'll find *Nnam-owondo*, a dish that dances in banana leaves or cooks directly in a pot. Picture this: grilled peanut paste, spiced up and slow-cooked, perfect for spreading on things or enjoying with tubers. Nuts and seeds combine vegetables in dishes such as *Ndole*, a Cameroonian national meal featuring boiled groundnut paste in a bitter leaf concoction. Nuts also find companionship with carbs, as seen in Central Africa's *Topsi banana*, where green banana takes the stage in a delightfully nutty and seedy flavor fiesta!

Ever heard of *Fumbwa*? It's a fantastic dish blending nuts with wild spinach. In Nigeria, they call those leaves Okazi, while in Cameroon, it's known as Eru or Nkok leaves. Now, let's hop over to Fiji for a taste adventure called *Ivi*, where grated chestnuts meet taro leaves and coconut milk, all wrapped up and steamed in banana leaves (version without sugar). It's like taking your taste buds on a delightful journey through different flavors!

That takes me back to the memories of holidays at our grandparents' farms! Now, let's be honest: digging up weeds wasn't exactly a thrill, but oh, the magic of harvesting made it all worthwhile. Picture this: pulling peanuts straight from the earth or yanking corn and having an impromptu taste test right then and there. But the real highlight was when we got back home! We gathered around a massive pot of *Coki*, *Condre*[14], or *Nkwa Nzap*[15], simmering away on a three-stone wood fire. And while the anticipation for that deliciousness built up, we'd throw corn or African pears on the fire, giving us some tasty appetizers to munch on.

---

[14] Condre is a traditional dish from West Cameroon, featuring green plantains, red palm oil, meat, hot pepper, and an array of spices, all cooked together to create a burst of flavor.

[15] Nkwa Nzap is a traditional dish from West Cameroon made with pounded cocoyam and sautéed huckleberry leaves.

The absolute joy, though, was in the lively conversations with our extended family and friends. Laughter filled the air as we swapped stories and enjoyed the simple pleasures of life. And hey, let's not forget those nuts – *Kola nuts*, for instance, were savored raw, though mainly by the grown-ups. Those were the days – good times, good food, and the warmth of shared moments!

Now let's shine a spotlight on a familiar face: African pears, also known as *Safou*, *Atanga*, or *Ube*. African pears are like nature's princesses—small, about 7 cm long, and rocking shades of blue or purple. They're not just pretty; they're a powerhouse of healthy fats. Indulging in a diet featuring delights like these pears not only treats us to amazing fats but also showers us with antioxidants, ensuring a protective shield for our overall health and heart. It's not just a snack; it's a flavor-packed journey for our well-being! Taste-wise, they're a delightful combo of tangy and sweet. Boiled or roasted, enjoyed solo or paired with roasted corn or plantain, it's a treat much like how you'd savor avocado. Nature's bounty sure knows how to keep things interesting!

When African pears take center stage during their season, they become the go-to street snack in West and Central African hotspots like Nigeria and Cameroon. Picture this: people roasting them on small, handmade barbecues, often alongside roasted corn cobs or ripe plantains. As the pears roast, they take on a dark, oily sheen, and when cracked open, they reveal a mouthwateringly rich and buttery flesh. It's a sight that makes your taste buds do a happy dance!

These snacks are a hit among those who skipped breakfast or need a quick pick-me-up during work breaks.

Animal fat source

Let's talk about animal fat, and no, it's not just about your regular meat cuts. We're talking about rich sources like dry and fresh fish, seafood, eggs, free-range chickens living their best lives, and even some bush meat. Now, when I think of free-roaming chickens, it reminds me of Dschang, the village where my parents settled after retiring, bringing back one of my favorite memories.

Back in those days, going to the village meant seeing my dad and late mom again. I miss you so much, Maman. Your beauty, your scent—I ache for the special spark in your eye when you looked at me. It spoke volumes of your boundless love without words. I miss the warmth it brought to my heart. Your absence has left an abyssal emptiness in me.

You see, my parents decided to trade city life for a serene village after a successful career in various towns in Cameroon. Interestingly their house is less than a 30-minute stroll away from my mother-in-law.

During one holiday, my husband, our four kids, and I took a trip to Dschang. Our oldest son had just turned 9, and our youngest daughter was still an infant at the time. It was during this holiday that they saw live chickens for the first time. Cue the excitement! They chased after every chicken in my mother-in-law's yard, pure joy on their faces. Ignoring her warnings, they kept playing until, oops, one of the chickens ended up in the pot sooner than planned that day. This particular chicken is known as the *Jungle chicken* in the Pacific Islands, *Village chicken*, or *Poulet bicyclette* depending on where you are in Africa. Trust me, they have a genuinely unmatched taste, an authentic real chicken flavor!

1.2.3. Proteins-rich food

Imagine our body as a lively community with a cast of thousands – proteins, each with a special talent!

Proteins are like our body's architects, ensuring everything from muscles to bones is in top shape and growing as it should. But proteins have even more tricks up their sleeve:

- ❖ Antibodies, our immune system's bodyguards, are proteins.
- ❖ Hemoglobin, which carries oxygen around our body, is made of proteins, ensuring oxygen gets to where it needs to go.
- ❖ Enzymes, our body's little helpers, speed up all kinds of beneficial reactions inside us.
- ❖ Most of our hormones, except for a few like sex hormones and the stress hormone cortisol, are proteins, too. They act as regulators, keeping everything from our mood to our metabolism running smoothly.

So yeah, proteins are pretty much involved in everything important going on in our bodies!

But here's the key: quality counts. For top-notch protein, stick to traditional foods to savor the full range of protein power.

Proteins hold a significant place in the traditional foods of tropical countries. The choice of protein sources depends on where people live and their way of life. They obtain protein from a variety of sources, including seafood, fish, bush meat, and meat from domesticated animals. Additionally, plant-based proteins like beans, chickpeas, lentils (dhal), and peas are commonly enjoyed. In certain regions, insects are even considered a delicacy. The variety in protein choices reflects what is available and ties in with the culinary tastes that are deep-rooted in the culture.

Plant-Based Protein Source

In many tropical countries, beans and lentils are a common and important part of people's diets. They come in all sorts of colors and types, like white, red, purple, striated, and black. Beans are fantastic for us because they're packed with fiber, vitamin K, potassium, magnesium, folate, iron, vitamin A, and loads of other vitamins, minerals, and antioxidants. Eating beans can help manage our blood pressure and blood sugar levels, and they're great for keeping our gut and nervous system healthy.

One popular type of bean in Africa is cowpeas, known as Niébé in the Sahel region. Cowpeas are a great source of plant-based protein and can even help with conditions like anemia because they are rich in iron and folic acid.

People in different places enjoy beans in traditional ways. For example, in the Caribbean, stewed red beans are very popular. In Cameroon, we make a dish called *Coki* by turning cowpeas into a paste. We mix it with taro leaves, red palm oil, salt, and some water, then wrap it in banana leaves and steam it until it's cooked. In Nigeria and Sierra Leone, they have similar dishes called *Moyi Moyi* and *Olélé*, but they add extra ingredients like eggs, crayfish, dry fish, and other seasonings. These meals are super yummy and nutritious.

You might wonder what makes food so unique when steamed in a banana leaf. It's the extra nutrients from the banana leaf that infuse into the food, giving it an unmatched flavor. This method results in a flavorful and highly nutritious meal while also preserving most of the nutrients. In West and Central Africa, people also make dishes by pounding beans with boiled plantains or potatoes (either Irish or sweet) and adding uncooked red palm oil. In Cameroon, it's called *Metita ncheu*[16] when made with potatoes or *Nkeding ncheu* with plantains.

These dishes take me on a trip down memory lane. I recall the joy of savoring Metita Ncheu right from the pot while my mom was still pounding it, steam wafting up. My important job then was tasting for salt, all while basking in my mom's indulgent gaze. By the time the meal reached the table, I was already satisfied—sheer bliss!" For those who prefer to keep their beans whole, another delicious option is to boil them, then sauté with tomatoes and spices for a tasty alternative.

Animal-based protein source

Imagine this culinary journey: in certain corners of the world, people craft mouthwatering meals using meat or fish, blending them with the rich flavors of palm oil or coconut oil and a medley of local spices. What sets this culinary masterpiece apart is the wrapping – they lovingly encase the concoction in banana leaves, steaming or slow-baking it in hot wood ashes. The

[16] Metita Ncheu is a West Cameroon delectable dish consisting of mashed potatoes and beans, enhanced with the rich and earthy flavor of red palm oil. When is cooked with plantain, it is called "Nkeding Ncheu".

result? A special dish called *Luwombo* in Uganda, *Ngweya* in Cameroon, or *Liboke* in Congo where the flavors dance with the addition of traditional oil.

Now, let's hop over to other African countries, particularly Yaoundé, Cameroon, where edible insects take center stage, with grasshoppers stealing the spotlight. You see, Every November, it's grasshopper season. They come together under the glow of streetlights, creating a magical halo as if straight from an artist's imagination. It's such a captivating scene; you might believe it's pure magic. During this season, people embark on the grasshopper hunt, armed with plastic bottles to fill. Yes, it takes hours, but it's not just a task – it's pure fun!

Here's a touching memory: my mom absolutely loved grasshoppers, and you know what? She was born in November. So, for her birthday, my brothers and I turned hunters, catching grasshoppers as a special gift. The best part? We'd present them to her at midnight while they were still lively in the container. The joy on her face was absolutely priceless. After a little prep work – wings and legs removed – we'd sauté the grasshoppers until they were crispy, creating a delightful dish that tasted surprisingly like seafood. And you bet I made sure to be around when she indulged so she could share the crunchy goodness. Now, that's a memory worth savoring!

In Africa and many tropical corners of the world, a whole insect banquet unfolds. Palm weevil grubs, caterpillars, termites, and grasshoppers take the stage. These little critters aren't just for show – they're packed with protein, fat, vitamins, and minerals, delivering a powerhouse punch to our immune systems and overall health. Whether enjoyed solo or paired with grains, tubers, or plantains, these protein and fat-rich meals are a tradition in many households.

And hey, it's not just the foods themselves that pack a nutritional punch. The way we preserve these traditional delights is another secret weapon, boosting the vitamin and mineral content. Intrigued? Stay tuned for the next topic—we're diving into the art of preserving traditional foods!

1.3. Traditional Food Preservation Techniques Boost Our Immune System

In Tropical countries, how people preserve food dates back to our ancestors. They were wise about nature and lived in harmony with it. To survive, they used what nature offered: the sun for drying, salt for dehydration, firewood for smoking, and fermentation. They didn't use harmful chemicals. Each method adds variety to our food choices and makes more nutrients available.

Fermentation

Embarking on a Pacific adventure, I decided to try my hand at making *Bobolo or Chikwangue*, a traditional Central African gluten-free bread crafted from fermented cassava. Little did I know that my kitchen would turn into a fragrant haven for three to four days. Now, some might find the aroma a bit off-putting, but to me, it was a comforting and thrilling reminder of home. Let's be honest, certain cheeses, such as camembert, could rival my bread in the scent department!

The journey to create *Bobolo* was no cakewalk—I had underestimated the effort involved. Yet, as the days passed and the fermentation magic worked its wonders, I couldn't help but feel a surge of pride. Gone were the days of haggling with the local seller over the price; now, I understood the true value of the labor involved. *Mintoumba* is another traditional bread that's popular in Cameroon. It's quite similar to *bobolo*, but with the addition of palm oil.

In tropical countries, fermentation extends beyond merely a culinary tradition; it becomes a way of life. Beyond preserving food and preventing waste, it increases nutrients, improves digestibility, and boosts dishes' longevity. These foods bring in a diverse team of good bacteria, turning our belly into a thriving ecosystem. Now, why does that matter? Well, a happy and varied good bacterial crew overpowers the harmful bacteria. The more good bacteria, the stronger our immune system.

Tropical countries are like the rock stars of fermented delights. The delicious foods we're about to explore pack a powerful nutritional punch.

Tubers-based fermentation

In many tropical countries, people have special dishes made from fermented cassava. Take *Bobolo*, for example. Its cooking process starts with fermenting cassava for a few days, then washing it with clean water to remove roots and excess liquid. After that, the flesh is finely mashed. This paste is then expertly wrapped in *Moi Moi leaves*, tied securely with thread, and steamed. In Fiji, they add a hint of sugar to this dish, turning it into a delightful dessert called *Bila*. Fermented cassava can also yield to *Water Fufu* or *Placali,* along with *Attieke* and *Gari*. *Attieke* and *Gari* are dried forms of fermented cassava, while *Water Fufu* is the wet form, creating a paste. In Fiji and the Pacific, they use a cool method called pit fermentation, especially for breadfruit. They peel and core the breadfruit, put it in a pit lined with leaves, cover it with more leaves and soil or rocks, and let it ferment for five to seven days. After that, they can cook the breadfruit at any time. The final product is washed, pounded, kneaded, and then cooked before eating.

Grains-based fermentation

In West-Central Africa, there's a dish called *Ogi*, also known as *Pap*, which is a fermented cereal pudding made from maize, sorghum or millet. Besides being rich in carbohydrates, corn is packed with fiber and minerals such as potassium and magnesium. This makes it a smart choice for maintaining heart health and stable blood sugar levels. Just keep an eye on the sugar content!

We also have *Fura*, which is like a wholesome hug in a bowl, crafted from fermented millet and enriched with nutritious milk. The millet is a special type of carb packed with protein, fiber, and antioxidants. Its fermentation boosts the availability and absorption of these nutrients, making *Fura* highly nutritious. It's great for your heart and helps prevent type 2 diabetes, among other health benefits. It's a burst of goodness!

Nuts and Seeds-based fermentation

Let's talk about a flavor-packed adventure in West African cuisine – nuts and seeds-based fermentation! Ever heard of *Ogiri*? It's made from fermented seeds like *Egusi*, and sesame. Pour this magic paste into your soups, and voila! Not only does it add an explosion of flavor, but it's also a probiotic powerhouse.

Now, meet the locust bean, also known as *Iru*, *Soumbala*, or *Niététou* in West Africa. Brace yourself for its bold aroma—some find it off-putting, while others call it intriguing. But hey, this little bean is a nutritional dynamo! Packed with fat, protein, calcium, fiber, and antioxidants, it's like a health power in disguise. Be sure to explore the recipe in Chapter 6!

Eating locust beans is a culinary escapade and a health trip. From preventing diabetes to tackling heart issues and colon cancer, this bean does it all.

Beverage-based fermentation

Let's take a sip into the world of beverage-based fermentation, where tradition meets taste and health!

First up on our journey is *Pito* from Northern Ghana – a powerhouse made from millet, guinea corn, or maize. Imagine an energy drink that's not only super refreshing but also a nutritional champ. *Pito* is loaded with essential minerals, giving your body the fuel it needs to grow and function at its best. Sip regularly, and you might just be waving diseases goodbye!

Now, let's swing over to Nigeria and Cameroon, where *Emu* and *Mbangui* (palm wine) are popular choices. Made by collecting sap from palm trees and letting it dance through the fermentation process, these drinks are rich in potassium, a friend to our body's well-being.

Shifting our focus to another delightful experience, we enter the world of Raffia palm wine, a beloved treasure enjoyed throughout Africa. Whether it's fermented or not, this beverage stands out as a champion. Bursting with essential nutrients, including powerful antioxidants, it emerges as a health hero, particularly benefiting those navigating the challenges of high blood sugar.

Dairy-based products

Meet *Wara*, the cool cousin of cheese, gracing plates across West Africa. How is it made? By giving milk a magical makeover—curdling it and separating the creamy parts with proteins and fats from the liquid parts with water and whey. It's like cheese's laid-back sibling but with all the flavor. Then there's *Kule Naoto*, the traditional fermented milk of the Maasai in Kenya, popular among people living in eastern Africa. In South Africa, we have *Amasi*, a traditional cream cheese made from sour milk and salt. *Ergo* is Ethiopia's take on yogurt, made from cow, camel, or goat's milk, depending on what's available.

These fermented milk products bring a joyful team of probiotics to our gut. So, whether you're savoring *Kule Naoto*, enjoying *Amasi*, or indulging in *Wara* and *Ergo*, you're treating your taste buds and caring for your gut!

However, while fermentation is fantastic for our health, it must be done correctly. If not, it can do more harm than good. The key to success lies in a few essential guidelines. Here's the lowdown on fermenting.

Fermentation basic tips

Seal the Deal: Cover your fermenting concoction like it's a secret potion. Whether it's a lid or a trusty cheesecloth, keeping the container tightly sealed wards off unwanted guests like mold, yeast, and pesky insects. You're aiming for good bacteria, not surprise contaminants.

Container Caution: Not all containers are created equal. Steer clear of metals like cast iron, copper, aluminum, and brass—they might throw an unexpected party with your food, causing off-flavors or strange color changes. Stick to the cool kids of the container world: glass or high-quality stainless steel.

Temperature Tango: Like a Goldilocks (a place that's not too hot and not too cold) situation, fermentation prefers the temperature to be just right. Too high, and harmful bacteria might crash the party, making you sick. Too low, and you'll be waiting forever for your fermented masterpiece. Aim for that sweet spot between 18 and 22 degrees Celsius—ideal for health benefits, flavor, and that oh-so-enticing aroma of the final product. Cheers to a fermentation journey without the hiccups!

Drying foods

Let's journey back in time and unravel the age-old art of drying food, a practice deeply rooted in the traditions of tropical places. Picture this: a bounty of fish, fruits, veggies, and more, but the challenge lies in consuming them before they go bad. Drying them out extends their edible lifespan.

This drying magic becomes especially invaluable during the "lean season." Think of it as the time when fresh produce is scarce because the crops are still basking in the sun, waiting to be harvested. When fresh food becomes a rare gem and prices soar, the brilliance of dried food shines through, offering a wallet-friendly alternative.

Fast-forward to today, and we've got nifty gadgets like ovens and food dryers, making the ancient practice of drying food a breeze. It's like a high-tech nod to our ancestors, a modern twist on a timeless technique that ensures our pantry stays stocked.

Smoking food

Let's take a flavorful journey into the world of smoking food—a tradition that's evolved from our ancestors' wild game-smoking days to a modern-day affair with chickens, pigs, cows, and seafood. Smoking is not just about preservation; it adds an incredible depth of flavor. Back in the day, our wise ancestors opted for hardwood for safety, and today, we're carrying on the tradition with a few upgrades.

In the vibrant culinary scenes of the Caribbean, Pacific, and Africa, smoked delights like crayfish and *Bounga*, *Ika*, or catfish are culinary superstars. Their smoky essence brings an irresistible umami taste to dishes, elevating them to a whole new level. The Caribbeans even have a gourmet delight called stewed smoked fish, adding a touch of elegance to the table.

Venture into West-Central Africa, where traditional dishes find their perfect match in the smoky embrace of smoked fish or meat. Think of delectable sauces like *Sauce Graine* from Côte d'Ivoire, mouthwatering dishes like *Ekwang* from Cameroon, not to mention the beloved *Egusi sauce* from West Africa. So, smoking isn't just a method for extending the life of food; it's a delicious twist that transforms ordinary dishes into extraordinary culinary experiences!

Salting food

Let's sprinkle some flavor on the art of preserving food with a dash of salt and a touch of sunshine! In the heart of Africa, this cherished tradition is a flavorful secret handed down through generations. Similarly, in the Pacific and Caribbean, the art of salting fish is often coupled with either drying or smoking.

But there's more to the story! Beyond preserving, these regions unveil a world of traditional cooking techniques that tantalize our taste buds and give a nod to our health. It's like a culinary journey where every sprinkle of salt and ray of sunshine brings out the best in our dishes and keeps our traditions alive and thriving!

Beyond preserving our favorite bites, traditional cooking techniques play a secret role in supporting our health. Let's unveil this culinary magic right now!

1.4. Traditional cooking techniques keep and enhance food antioxidants content

Foods that are charred, fried, over-grilled, over-roasted or seared, especially meats cooked at high temperatures, can produce AGEs (Advanced Glycation End Products). Those foods taste amazing! But, like a double-edged sword, they can also seriously harm our health. The more heat and browning, the more AGEs you get, which can mess with your immune system, cause chronic diseases, and speed up aging.

Processed foods, fast food, aged cheese, and meat from hormone and grain-fed animals are also packed with Ages. The food industry has even found ways to produce and add AGEs to food to enhance flavor.

Luckily, you can cut down on AGEs by drinking teas such as moringa tea, green tea, honeybush tea, and eating traditional foods including avocado, *Safu*, nuts and seeds, parsley, celery, veggies, fruits, and spices. Also, cooking methods like slow cooking, boiling, stewing, steaming, gentle grilling, or baking keep more nutrients in your food without loading it with AGEs.

Earth oven, dirt oven

In some Tropical countries, people have a cool way of cooking called an earth oven. In Samoa, it's called *Umu*, for the Maori people in New Zealand, it's *Hangi*, and in Fiji, they call it *Lovo*. In the Pacific Islands, it is men's business. The guys usually take charge of this cooking method. Maybe it's because it involves digging a hole in the ground? Whatever the case, after the hole is created, they partially fill it with stones and set a fire. Once the flames have subsided, the food is wrapped in coconut and breadfruit leaves, layered with several more leaves, and left to cook in the oven created by the makeshift earth pit for a few hours. This gives the food a smoky, delicious taste. In certain Caribbean countries such as Trinidad and Tobago, a traditional "dirt oven" is made from soil and clay right on the ground. It functions like a modern oven, and they use it to bake various foods, including bread.

In West Africa, there's a cooking method that imparts a smoky flavor by wrapping food in banana leaves and slow-cooking it under hot ash. Absolutely delicious!

Transitioning to Fiji, where I lived, there were construction projects near my house. I befriended the workers, and they shared their plan to cook *Lovo* for the first Easter after Covid-19. Excited, I asked if I could join them, and they happily agreed. They even suggested bringing any food I wanted to cook in the earth oven.

On the anticipated day, I simply crossed the road to where they had dug a hole in the middle of a banana plantation. Concerned about the banana trees, I voiced my worry, but the workers assured me it would be fine, and I trusted their judgment. And so, that's how I found myself helping to make *Lovo* for the first time.

For the feast, I contributed yams, while they brought meat and taro leaves for *Palusami*, a delightful Fijian delicacy featuring taro leaves, tuna fish, and coconut milk. Using coconut shells, they prepared the *Palusami*, which I paired with my yams. Sharing this flavorful meal with my daughter, I expressed gratitude to my newfound friends for the wonderful experience. It felt as though Lovo had come right to my home, saving me the journey yet offering an enriching encounter!

Steaming food in palm and banana leaves

In traditional cooking practices in tropical regions, people commonly utilize bananas and palm leaves. These leaves are used to wrap food, which is then slowly steamed or baked. The distinct taste imparted to the food is attributed to the presence of a specific type of antioxidant found in the leaves. Although we don't consume the leaves themselves, they generously release antioxidants into the food during the cooking process, enhancing its taste and nutritional value. It's truly remarkable to acknowledge the ingenuity of our ancestors to discover an effective way to promote both the healthiness and enjoyment of our food!

Boiling

When we talk about boiling, it means cooking with water, where the liquid covers the food. Tubers such as cassava, yams, and sweet potatoes are frequently boiled, a process that helps eliminate antinutrients and enhances the overall digestibility of the food.

Soaking before cooking

Soaking is like giving grains and legumes a little bath, making them more digestible by breaking down antinutrients and other substances that can be tough on our gut. It makes it easier for our bodies to absorb essential nutrients. This age-old trick has proven to be quite beneficial!

For instance, soaking beans, lentils, peas, and cowpeas (black-eyed peas or *Niébé*) overnight for about 15 hours reduce their cooking time and increase vital nutrients like fibers, aiding in improved digestion. A simple water drain once or twice is all it takes. This soaking process also reduces gas-producing sugars, sparing us from bloating and any unintended awkward moments when our bodies release noisy gas.

Here are some soaking tips:

1. Soak your beans, peas, cowpeas or lentils overnight. When it's time to cook them, add some salt and two teaspoons of apple cider vinegar for every kilogram of legume, but make sure to do this towards the end of cooking. If you add the salt too soon, it'll slow down the cooking time. The apple cider vinegar really helps, especially after soaking, as it breaks down the sugars that cause gas, making those legumes easier to digest.

2. For grains like rice, corn, millet, and sorghum, you get the best nutrients after soaking. Cover the grains with enough water, and add a bit of whey (from dairy), lemon juice, or apple cider vinegar. Then, cover it tightly and let it soak overnight (or up to 24 hours).

Even though our traditional food provides a diverse range of options, it would be such a shame not to explore the culinary offerings of other cultures.

2. Key Guidelines for Tropical Foods

Like any nutritious and healing food, tropical food has guidelines to follow. Just because you're eating your traditional food doesn't mean you're automatically protected. You need to follow these guidelines to get the best out of it:

Portion size is crucial: Have you ever noticed the plates at African, Caribbean, and Pacific Islander events? They're often piled so high with food that it's a struggle to carry them without spilling! The leftovers are equally impressive, and those who actually manage to finish their plates can barely move afterward.

Some of these foods are high in tropical oils that make everything taste so scrumptiously delicious! Let's be real—who would eat a pale *Coki (Moi Moi)* or *Fumbwa* instead of one that's red-orange and green-red? Or *Egusi* sauce, *Afang* without that reddish touch of red palm oil? I'm not saying to go heavy on the oils, but using the right amount makes our food delicious. After all, family meals are meant to be shared among family members, unless you decide to go solo and overindulge. The problem here is the portion size.

When you overeat, it puts a lot of pressure on your digestive system, making your stomach expand beyond normal. Your body quickly lets you know it's not happy with this treatment. You feel tired, sluggish, and need a long rest to recover. Even your clothes become tighter in protest. If this happens at dinner time, you'll likely have trouble sleeping too. So, just because Tropical food is healing doesn't mean you can overeat.

Now, I bet you're wondering what the right amount of food is for you. The short answer? Your body knows best. There's no one-size-fits-all answer but starting the habit of serving smaller portions can help you pay attention to when your body is satisfied. This is mindfulness. Once you start eating mindfully, you'll get in tune with your body. This creates a win-win where your body gets what it needs, and you can fully enjoy the benefits of this traditional food.

Proportions matter too: African, Caribbean, and Pacific Islander plates are usually full of carbs, with barely any other types of food, and veggies are almost nonexistent. This imbalance can upset your body, leading to constipation, bloating, weight gain, and other health issues. Even a high-carb diet needs balance on the plate.

Variety matters: Traditional food works best when part of a well-rounded meal. Each traditional food shines when paired with other foods. For example, eating cassava with sautéed greens provides more health benefits than eating cassava alone. Having carbs, fats, proteins, and lots of veggies on your plate is just the combo your body need to thrive.

The real magic happens when you mix things up! Instead of sticking to just rice, yam or *Chikwangue*, switch it up with sweet potatoes, plantains, maize, cassava or millet based on what's locally available. If carrots are your go-to veggie, try adding in some greens, red veggies like cabbage, or yellow ones like peppers for a pop of color. Love your meat? Awesome! But don't forget to bring in beans, cowpeas, and lentils for variety. And if you're all about that red palm oil, fantastic—but try blending it with groundnut, coconut, or olive oil too. Your body craves variety to unlock a wider range of benefits!

Watch out for the processed versions of traditional foods: Many people living abroad go for convenience and choose processed versions of their traditional foods. For example, processed palm oil may have a colorless appearance that appeals to some people, but our bodies know it is harmful.

Take your time when eating: Why rush through your meals? Isn't it supposed to be an enjoyable time? Eating is your time and deserves more attention. Eating slowly treats your body with the respect and care it deserves, allowing for better digestion and utilization of the food you eat.

3. Don't get Bored With Your Traditional Food. Get creative

Mealtime is genuinely delightful, something people eagerly anticipate every day. However, having the same food with identical flavors can become monotonous, right? Let's spice things up and infuse creativity into our meals to keep things interesting. We can achieve this in two ways:

Get Flexible with Your Traditional Foods

Ready to shake things up with our traditional favorites? Let's talk about the magic of flexibility in our beloved dishes. I absolutely love our traditional food—the rich aroma, the spice-filled warmth, and that unique, familiar taste that brings comfort.

But here's the thing – have you ever dared to swap out a key ingredient and see what happens? Picture this: leafy greens sautéed in palm oil. It's a flavor explosion that feels like a warm hug. Now, try it with a different oil – still good, but undeniably different. The beauty lies in the unexpected, and you won't know until you give it a shot.

When the idea of juggling multiple dishes feels like a bit much, why not blend them into one glorious, balanced creation? I've tried this with various dishes like tomato stew, okra sauce, fried rice, butter chicken, and curry sauce. For example, adding taro leaves or locally grown greens to Coki or Moyi Moyi really elevates the experience. The secret? The more veggies, the better! Whether it's okra, Egusi, or curry sauce, tossing in green leafy goodness makes the dish shine. Picture a hearty potato stew with a burst of chopped veggies or the perfect blend of broccoli and leafy greens in a tantalizing Yassa (onion sauce). Just reminiscing about these mouthwatering creations has me ready to hit the kitchen!

Borrow ideas from other culinary cultures.

Let's buckle up for a culinary adventure!

First things first, let's break free from our bubble and dive into the delightful world of mixing things up. Have you ever thought about borrowing flavors from other cultures ? It's like a magic trick—turning ordinary meals into exciting, enjoyable experiences. Because, let's face it, the joy of food lies in its ever-changing, ever-surprising nature!

Now, let's take a detour and talk about borrowing ideas from other culinary cultures. Thanks to globalization, our kitchens have become gateways to the world. All we need is a phone and the internet, and we can virtually taste the globe through social media and YouTube. I've stumbled upon some incredible recipes just by hitting play on a YouTube video. Sure, some were kitchen triumphs, and others, well, not so much. But hey, the adventure is in the exploration!

As we journey through the global kitchen, the true enchantment reveals itself when we engage with food enthusiasts from various corners of the globe. Take, for example, my friend from Russia, who introduced me to the delightful fusion of flavors in Solyanka, creating a rich tapestry of tastes that transcends borders. Thanks to her, I've unlocked the secret recipe for the sour and salty Solyanka, a lip-smacking Russian soup (check out the recipe section) featuring ingredients readily available in tropical countries – meat, mushrooms, chicken, and veggies.

One of the things I find super cool is experimenting with ingredients. For example, I tried making dairy-free butter chicken by using coconut oil instead of butter. And the results ? The difference is hardly noticeable! Coconut oil, with its gentle flavor, makes an awesome alternative to butter.

Let's have fun trying out grains from different places, like quinoa. It's a South American plant that's known for being a complete source of plant-based protein. We can also explore the amazing world of Indian food, where lots of spices can add different flavors to what we eat. And hey, why not change up recipes from the West by using local ingredients? Like making a quiche with cassava flour and swapping bacon for soaked dried meat. And don't forget about Japanese tofu – it's full of plant protein and can be used in lots of different ways in our cooking, including in lieu of meat in sauces. Let's stay in Japan and discover the wonders of Asian seaweed. This versatile, age-old tradition can be a game-changer in our kitchen. Whether enjoyed alone or in soups, it is a secret weapon for those who fancy their stock cubes. Say goodbye to MSG side effects – seaweed provides natural glutamate, the umami magic we're all seeking, into the stock cubes. It's not just fantastic flavor; it's a nutrient powerhouse, packed with minerals, antioxidants, and iodine that promote thyroid health.

Forget about the synthetic iodine in table salt, which our body does not absorb as well as the natural one – dive into the natural goodness of seaweed. It's like a supercharged boost that our bodies love to soak up. Take brown seaweed, for example, like the fabulous wakame. Brace yourself because it packs a punch – 13.5 times the antioxidant power of vitamin E! Talk about a nutrient powerhouse.

But that's not all—seaweed is our go-to for a fiber fiesta. And the perks don't stop there—it's got this fantastic trio of anti-inflammatory, anti-cancer, and anti-diabetic properties. Who knew a humble sea plant could be so powerful?

Just make sure you choose organic seaweed to avoid heavy metal exposure from ocean pollution. Also, keep an eye on the salt content—it can be a bit salty. The options for seaweed choice are numerous, but for the most nutritious punch, go for the brown seaweed: kelp, wakame, fucus, hijiki, and kombu.

So, are you ready to unleash your inner culinary explorer? It's time to mix, match, and savor the world, one delicious bite at a time!

Now, moving on to the next stop in my SET-FREE method – it's fasting! Let's zoom in on this intriguing practice, especially after discovering the incredible healing powers of our traditional foods. Are you curious to explore the benefits of fasting and uncover the secrets it holds for our well-being? Let's dig in!

B. Fasting

Fasting is the greatest remedy - the physician within Philippus Paracelsus- 1493-1541
-Swiss physician

1. Is Fasting Another Trending Diet?

Have you caught wind of the fasting buzz lately? It's the talk of the town, and everyone's tuning in! Fasting, an age-old tradition for well-being, has made a serious comeback and is stealing the spotlight in discussions about staying healthy in Western countries. It's like the ancient secret to a modern-day health kick!

Now, you might be thinking, "Is fasting just another trendy diet in the mix of all these new ones?" With all the diet crazes out there, it's easy to think fasting is just about dropping those extra pounds. But it's way more than that. Fasting is a lifestyle that's been around for over 2.5 million years—yeah, that's ancient history! Back then, our hunter-gatherer ancestors would feast after a successful hunt and then go without food until the next big catch. That was their way of life, balancing times of plenty with times of scarcity. It's fascinating to think that our bodies have been wired for fasting for such a long time.

Fast forward to about 10,250 years ago, and bam! Agriculture entered the scene, changing how we eat. Then, 250 years ago, the industrial era brought another wave of change. But despite all these shifts, our bodies have this ancient memory of fasting ingrained in them—about 2.5 million years' worth, to be exact.

In today's world, we find ourselves on a journey to embrace new ways of living and eating. This isn't an instant change; it's more like giving our body a software update. So, be patient—it might take a bit of time, perhaps even as much as 2.5 million years to adjust to our modern life eating habits. In the meantime, our bodies are still tuned into the fasting memory, ready to reward us when we practice fasting.

Throughout history, many religions and ancient traditions—Buddhism, Christianity, Islam, Judaism, Taoism, Jainism, and Hinduism—have embraced fasting to connect the body and mind. Even super-smart people like Pythagoras, the math whiz from Ancient Greece, used to fast before exams to make their brains supercharged. Pythagoras, the brilliant mind from Ancient Greece, embarked on a 40-day fast and was amazed to find that it not only heightened his brainpower but also contributed to increased physical strength. So impressed was he by the benefits that he enthusiastically shared his experience with his students, encouraging them to give it a try for themselves. Other wise thinkers like Hippocrates, Socrates, Plato, Aristotle, and monks also believed in fasting for both feeling good in the body and thinking clearly in the mind.

Now, as fasting's health benefits make a comeback, scientists are diving deep into it, eager to unlock its secrets. The excitement peaked in 2016 when the Japanese scientist Yoshinori Ohsumi bagged a Nobel Prize in Medicine. What did he find? Something called autophagy.

Autophagy serves as the superpower inherent in our cells, acting as their mechanism for housecleaning, healing, and providing our bodies with an invigorating internal makeover. What sparks this incredible process? Fasting and extended exercise! For now, let's focus on fasting. When we choose to skip a meal or two, our bodies seamlessly transition into autophagy mode, independently addressing and repairing issues without requiring any external assistance.

Now, let's break it down. Imagine your body as a busy worker with loads of tasks. Every time you munch on something, it's like handing your organs another assignment. But just like how you need a breather from work, your organs need a timeout from processing food. And that's where fasting swoops in.

During a fast, our organs get a break, and that's when the magic happens. They start repairing and refreshing our body's cells, like hitting the reset button for our health. This process lowers insulin levels and blood pressure, among other health benefits.

In a nutshell, fasting is like a break that keeps our bodies in tip-top shape. So, the next time you think about skipping a meal, just remember – you're giving your body a chance to heal!

2. The Relationship Between Fasting and Insulin Levels

As mentioned earlier, insulin is the elephant in the room of our health. Its job is to protect our body from harm when there's too much sugar in our blood. Just like firefighters, insulin quickly clears the extra sugar and sends it to our liver, muscles, and pancreas cells to keep our vital organs safe. If we continue to eat and take in a lot of sugary food, the cells might rebel against insulin and stop cooperating. This will lead to our body pumping out a lot of insulin to force the blood sugar into the cells. This is a condition called insulin resistance. As the cells close themselves, insulin goes on strike against us and start storing sugars in fat cells that are more welcoming. The initial signal is putting on weight, especially around our belly. If we ignore these warnings and let the fat accumulate, it can cause more severe health issues, including Type 2 diabetes, cardiovascular diseases, and certain types of cancer, as clearly illustrated in Figure 1.

Did you know that all food you eat affects insulin production? Yep! They just stimulate insulin production differently. For example, sugary drinks and processed foods can cause a quick spike in blood sugar and insulin levels because they often contain added sugar and lack enough fiber to slow down sugar absorption. On the other hand, foods rich in healthy fats like butter, oils, avocados, African pears, nuts, and seeds lead to a more balanced insulin release. Proteins from sources like beans, meat, and fish can make insulin levels rise a bit more than fats, but they still contribute to a healthy balance.

Insulin plays a key role in managing body weight, working like a double-edged sword. If you have too much insulin, you can gain weight and increase your risk of type 2 diabetes. On the other hand, if you have too little insulin, like in type 1 diabetes, you tend to be leaner. This shows how important insulin is for our weight and health. So, keeping insulin levels in check is important for controlling weight and staying healthy.

As you can see, fasting is like a multi-targeted metabolic therapy that can do many things for our bodies. It's a powerful tool that lowers insulin, preventing and reversing by then several chronic diseases induced by high levels of insulin. It helps us stay fit and even makes us smarter, younger, and slimmer. It's like giving our body 5-star care! Plus, it's free, easy, and doesn't require medicine, which might not thrill businesses like big pharma companies that profit when people are unwell.

3. The Clear Benefits of Fasting for Your Health

"A little starvation can really do more for the average sick man than can the best medicines and the best doctors."

Mark Twain

"I fast for greater physical and mental efficiency"

Plato

Lose Weight: Getting Your Ideal Body

As you fast, your body gracefully unveils its true shape, enhancing your appearance to cultivate a stunning and healthy physique. Fasting is a celebration of your body's innate ability to sculpt itself into a work of art. You will look like no one else but the finest and sexiest version of your striking self.

And if you've already achieved your desired weight, fear not. During fasting, your body recognizes this achievement, opting to utilize only minimal fat storage. It's like your body's way of saying, "I've got this. Let's maintain this fantastic physique together." So, embrace the journey of fasting as a pathway to unveil and celebrate the masterpiece that is your body.

Your Body Gets More Energy Options!

As you get older, your body struggles more with handling carbs and sugars. Fasting, whether short or long, helps your body learn to use both stored fat and glucose for energy. This boosts your "metabolic flexibility," which is like having extra power options. Think of it like the new MacBook Pro – it can charge with USB type-c or a magnetic charger. If one doesn't work, the other kicks in as a backup, making the MacBook more durable. Similarly, having the choice between glucose and fat for energy makes your body stronger, helping you resist and fight diseases. It's like giving your body a versatile and robust energy setup!

Makes New Brain Cells: Keeping Your Brain Healthy!

Fasting isn't just great for your body; it's a fantastic brain boost, too! When you fast, it improves your memory, makes learning easier, and keeps your brain super sharp.

Ever heard of BDNF (Brain-Derived Neurotrophic Factor)? It's a brain protein that gets a big boost during fasting. BDNF helps your brain cells grow, multiply, and stay strong against sickness. Activating BDNF during fasting is like giving your brain the power to form new connections and repair itself, similar to recovering from something like a stroke. So, fasting isn't just about skipping meals; it's also giving your brain the opportunity to be at its very best!

When your brain lacks enough BDNF, it might age faster and become more susceptible to illnesses like Parkinson's or Alzheimer's.

But here's the fascinating part: fasting, like during Ramadan, can make your brain produce more BDNF—up to 3.5 times more! It's like a special treat that gives your brain extra power to stay healthy. Isn't that tempting enough to do a Ramadan all year round?

New gene expression: you make more protein!

Your body starts from a tiny cell and it's pretty amazing how they grow into all the different parts, like organs, skin, hair, limbs, and so on. This process, which involves the creation of new protein, is called gene expression, where each part is customized to fit your body's needs. Even though every cell has the same genes, only some of them are active, and the rest are inactive.

The traits we usually notice, such as skin color or height, come from these active genes. But there's a lot happening behind the scenes – the active genes are like bosses, telling your cells what to do, like making new cells. Now, think about this: fasting can increase the number of active genes, giving your cells more opportunities to adapt and affecting how you recover from things like strokes or injuries. It's like giving your cells a little extra help to stay healthy!

Activates antioxidants genes: You get more antioxidants!

If you want your body to have a bunch of vitamins, minerals, and antioxidants, fasting can help with that! You don't need to buy fancy supplements, just try fasting! It gives your body a boost of antioxidants, which are like tiny protectors.

And that's not all – fasting activates special genes that reduce inflammation, helping your cells stay strong. Amazing, right?

Autophagy: your body's cleaning system gets activated!

Did you know your body has a cleaning system called autophagy? It helps you get rid of old, worn-out cells that can make you sick, making room for brand-new, super-strong, and healthier ones! In other words, autophagy heals. What's even more exciting is that fasting, which helps trigger autophagy, does this without any icky side effects like some medicines have. Autophagy is like a doctor inside you, and it doesn't ask for money—just a break from eating all the time!

Experts suggest that your body's cleaning system usually kicks in after 18 to 24 hours of not eating. Autophagy's peak time, is different for everyone and can be around 48 to 72 hours, which is like 2 to 3 days of fasting. So, giving your body a little break from eating for that long can really allow autophagy to do its fantastic cleaning job!

Stem Cell Mobilization: Your Body's Repair Crew

Think of stem cells as body repair workers originating from our bone marrow. When you resume eating after fasting, it's the moment for your body to swap out damaged cell parts cleared during autophagy. At this stage, the body signals stem cells to go to these cells and fix the damaged parts, but it typically takes about two to three days of water-only fasting for these stem cells to kick into action.

If you think three days of fasting sounds tough, consider this: buying stem cells is pricey, and there's no guarantee they'll work correctly. They will more likely end up in the wrong place, like hiring workers to fix your head but they mistakenly go to your heart. Are you thinking of using someone else's stem cells? Well, those cells might see your cells as strangers and start attacking them, confusing your body's defense system. Your body fully trusts only its own stem cells.

Speeding up your Metabolism: The Secret to Burn Fat

Guess what happens when you hit the pause button on eating? Your body doesn't slow down—it actually revs up! Think of your body as a car, and fasting is like giving it a little turbo boost. Once you've fasted for 48 hours, your body's engine, also known as metabolism, kicks into overdrive—it speeds up by a whopping 3.6 times! It's like hitting a reset button that leaves you feeling fresh and renewed.

If you go without eating for four days, the energy your body uses when you're just chilling or resting shoots up by a staggering 14%! So, fasting isn't a shutdown for your body; it's more like a supercharge that increases your metabolism. Who knew skipping a meal could make you feel so energized and alive?

Producing Growth Hormones: The Secret to Youth and Strong Muscles

Kids and teens tend to produce enough growth hormones to grow properly. When there's a shortage of these hormones, kids might end up a bit shorter than their peers. As for adults, the story changes – growth hormones tend to drop, resulting in lower muscle and bone mass, extra belly fat, and higher levels of bad cholesterol and triglycerides. But a bit of fasting can turn things around by increasing growth hormones that burn fat, make you look younger, and boost testosterone for building muscle.

Fasting for just two days can skyrocket the amount of these growth hormones in your body – we're talking about a fivefold increase! The real magic happens between two to three days of fasting, making you not just healthy but super strong too.

Now, I get it – some folks are all about shortcuts and might consider fake growth hormones via injections. But, that path can lead to issues like diabetes, high blood pressure, joint and muscle pain. So, why not stick to the natural boost from fasting? It's the real deal without side effects to deal with.

Prevent and reverse high insulin and some heart and metabolic diseases.

If you're looking to reverse metabolic and heart diseases, think of fasting as your medicine. Just like you wouldn't stop taking your meds when your blood pressure or insulin levels improve, you need to stick with fasting to keep those chronic diseases at bay.

I've helped people from all around the world get healthier through fasting—it's like a fun challenge for their bodies! After a few months of fasting, I noticed some awesome things happening. People lost weight, and their bodies got better at handling sugar. Even the tricky stuff like bad cholesterol and triglycerides went down! And people with high blood pressure saw improvements, too!

But that's not all. Some also reported that Fasting makes them feel happier and more confident and even boosts their libido. Plus, their heart health improved, as did their sleep quality and mental sharpness.

Insulin resistance

Insulin resistance usually comes from eating too many processed foods and snacking too often, making it a diet-related issue. Since type 2 diabetes and some heart issues are caused by insulin resistance, they're also tied to diet and need dietary changes. Fasting can help fix insulin resistance because it naturally lowers blood sugar and insulin levels without needing medication.

High blood pressure

Fasting lowers high blood pressure by lowering insulin.

Let's break down and simplify the connection between insulin and blood pressure:

Normally, a key player in your arteries called Nitric Oxide helps maintain healthy blood pressure. However, high insulin levels weaken that key player. When insulin levels go up, blood vessels narrow as the arteries' key player weakens, which can cause high blood pressure.

Here's where fasting comes in. Your insulin levels drop when you fast, and your arteries' key player increases and strengthens. As a result your blood pressure lowers and comes back to normal. Think of it like a seesaw—when insulin goes down, your blood pressure has a better chance of going down, too. So, fasting can be a great way to keep your blood pressure in check!

High cholesterol, High Triglycerides

Fasting reduces troublesome cholesterol and triglyceride levels by lowering insulin levels.

You have triglycerides and two types of cholesterol—the good one (HDL) and the not-so-good one (LDL). When you fast, insulin levels decrease, allowing a cleanup crew to clear your blood vessels. Fasting helps lower the LDL and triglycerides, which are like troublemakers causing heart problems.

At the same time, fasting boosts your HDL—it's like having more bodyguards to protect your heart! This matters because if your triglyceride to HDL ratio is off, it can lead to serious heart problems like atherosclerosis, stroke, and heart attacks.

So, fasting is like giving your heart a helping hand to stay strong and healthy.

The "When to eat" and "What to eat" questions are important, but "When" is seriously underappreciated

- Dr. Jason Fung, nephrologist. Toronto-Canada

4. Exploring Different Approaches to Fasting

Fasting might seem intimidating at first, but you might already be doing it without even realizing it. Remember those times when you were too busy at work to eat lunch or running late and skipped breakfast? That's fasting! The only difference is that it's unconscious. However, here I want to make fasting something you're aware of so you can personalize this lifestyle choice and choose what works best for you. Fasting can be as easy as missing a meal or two during the day or going without food for a longer period. The aim is to discover a fasting routine that fits your lifestyle—every fasting type, whether short or long, offers significant health benefits.

The table below describes some options to choose from. A combination of options is also a great idea.

Table 3: Overview of types and fasting options

Fasting type	Fasting options	Description	Approximate duration Of the fast
Short fasts	Intermittent fasting	This is short daily fasts. Eat your first meal at noon after a 12-hour fast, or have your meal anytime in the afternoon after fasting for 13 to 23 hours.	12H - 23H
Long fasts	Periodic Fasting	Fast 1-2 days. Meaning no food for 1 to 2 consecutives days. You can make it weekly, biweekly or monthly depending on your needs.	24H-48H
	Alternate day fasting	Skip a day of eating. Eat the next day. Make it weekly, biweekly, monthly depending on your needs.	36-40H
	Longer fasts	Complete a fast lasting more than two days. Do this quarterly, biannually, or as needed. This means not eating for more than two consecutive days..	Water fast for two days or more
Note: Throughout the fasting duration, stick to plain water, unsweetened tea, or coffee.			

For many people I've worked with, skipping breakfast tends to be simpler because not everyone feels hungry in the morning. Many who do eat breakfast are often in a rush and end up having a quick meal they barely enjoy. On the other hand, skipping dinner can be tougher for some since it's usually a time for family meals. You get to pick which meal is easier for you to skip and give it a try.

12-hour fast: A 12-hour fast simply means that if you have dinner at 7 pm, your breakfast should be around 7 am the next day. Likewise, if you have breakfast at 7 am, dinner should be around 7 pm.

16-hour fast: A 16-hour fast means that if you have dinner at 7 pm, your next meal, which would typically be lunch, should be around 11 am the next day.

23-hour fast: Imagine tailoring your fasting schedule to suit your favorite meal. If dinner is your highlight, start your 23-hour fast by enjoying a hearty meal at 7 pm, and the next day, relish dinner again at 6 pm. For those who cherish lunchtime, a satisfying meal at 1 pm kicks off your fast, with lunch the following day at 12 pm. And if breakfast is your thing, begin your day with a delicious meal at 9 am, and ensure your next morning's breakfast is ready by 8 am.

Longer fasts: Before you try a longer fast, it's a good idea to get used to shorter ones first.

Fasting varies from person to person, so it's all about figuring out what suits you best!

5. Caution on Who Should Fast

Are you thinking of trying fasting? It's usually fine for most people. But just like any medicine has its own info leaflet, fasting is a natural remedy with its own manual. This guide explains its benefits, different types for various conditions, and important precautions. Here are some key points to keep in mind.

Health Conditions and Medication: If you're not feeling well or taking meds, talk to your doctor before diving into fasting. They can give personalized advice, keep an eye on your health, and adjust prescriptions if needed.

Mental Health Concerns: If you are dealing with mental health stuff like depression or eating disorders, it's safer to skip fasting unless supervised by a nutritionist, dietitian, or therapist. Fasting could make mental health issues worse.

Underweight or Menstrual Irregularities: If you're underweight, especially if you're a young woman, having too little body fat can mess with your periods and make it tougher to get pregnant.

Pregnancy and Breastfeeding: Are you expecting or nursing? You need extra nutrients for yourself and your baby. It doesn't mean you should stuff yourself and eat all the time. Instead, it means there is a way to navigate fasting while still eating enough. You can have your usual two to three balanced meals and go easy on the snacks. Even with cravings, being mindful of what you eat will likely keep your pregnancy healthy.

Fasting too much: Doing long fasts too often or for too long (your body will let you know your limits) is like overdoing it at the gym. While both fasting and exercise are great for wellness, pushing them to extremes can backfire. Just as intense workouts can lead to injuries, prolonged fasting can stress your body and potentially cause more harm than good. Think of elite athletes who suffer from joint or muscle injuries due to overtraining. Similarly, taking fasting to an uncompromising level can be detrimental to your health. The key is to start slowly, see how your body reacts, and make adjustments as needed.

Simple Tips for Intermittent Fasting (Less Than 24 Hours)

Ready to kickstart intermittent fasting? Good news – you can start anytime you feel up for it! For a smoother start, consider cutting down on sugar a few days before diving in. The rules during and after intermittent fasting? They're pretty much like the ones for longer fasting – simple and effective!

Simple Tips for Longer Fasts (24 Hours and Beyond):

Whether fasting for 24 hours or 48 hours or even considering going without food for more than two days, take it step by step. Start with shorter fasts and see how your body reacts before trying longer ones. Let's begin with a 24-hour fast, then skip a day and assess your body's reaction before thinking about fasting for two days or more. It's all about practicing and learning to listen to your body's signals to find what works best for you on your fasting journey. After all, your body knows best.

Now, if you're itching to explore the wonders of extended fasting, I've got some tips to turn your journey into a breeze:

Preparing for Fasting

Two Weeks Before Fasting: Trim down on carbs, say goodbye to sugary treats, and add more healthy fats to your plate. This step will help your body ease into fasting and make the experience more comfortable.

Don't Stock Up: Skip the heavy meals right before starting your fast. Loading up on food just before fasting can make it more challenging for your body to adjust during the fasting period.

For Women Doing Long Fasts: Ladies, target the first two weeks of your period when estrogen is high—it makes fasting a bit easier. The next two weeks leading up to your next period might pose a challenge since progesterone is high, potentially bringing more hunger and snack cravings.

During fasting

- Hydrate Right: If you experience dizziness, lightheadedness, or a dry mouth while fasting, it could be a sign of dehydration. Remember to drink regularly, choosing plain water, tea, or coffee without sugar or milk to keep dehydration at bay. Plus, the polyphenols in teas can even help tackle the toxins your gut releases during fasting.

- Battle fasting hunger: It's normal to feel hungry while fasting, but remember, hunger comes and goes. Drinking water and tea helps ease hunger pangs. If you need an extra boost, you can get your favorite tea and add in some cinnamon, ginger, and lemon for additional flavor and appetite control. If that's not enough, you can also try "fat coffee," to keep hunger at bay. It is a tip from Dr. Jason Fung, a Canadian kidney and diet expert. Mix in a teaspoon of fats like coconut oil, red palm oil, or butter. These fats won't mess with your body's fat-burning mode. But watch out – introducing any sugar to your coffee can derail the fat-burning process, bidding farewell to your fasting perks! And remember, milk in coffee? Nope, that'll slam the brakes on the autophagy process. Stick to fats – no carbs, no protein – for fasting triumph!

- Cramp Relief: If fasting gives you cramps or headaches, try using magnesium. You can apply it as a cream or gel, or add a pinch of salt to your water. Epsom salt and magnesium sulfate crystals are also great options.

- Knowing when to halt your fasting journey is essential: The golden rule is to tune in to your body's cues while fasting. Fasting isn't always a smooth ride; some days are easier than others, just like in life. Both good and tough days are okay as long as you listen to and trust your body. It's highly recommended to stop fasting if:

You feel fatigued during fasting, your body might be signaling that you need to stop. However, tiredness can sometimes be mistaken for hunger. The psychological aspect of fasting can also be draining, but it's often manageable. You're the best judge of whether you can push through or if it's time to call it quits.

You're feeling queasy, throwing up, or your cramps and headaches just won't quit; it's like your body's way of saying, 'Hey, maybe it's time to stop fasting for now'.

Something else doesn't feel right, it's essential to stop and consult your healthcare provider before continuing.

You miss periods (women obviously!) during fasting. It could also indicate a need to pause and seek professional advice. Trust your body's signals and prioritize your well-being above all else.

After fasting

Once you've wrapped up your fast, here's the game plan:

- Start Slow: Ease back into eating with something light, like coconut water or bone broth (check out the recipe in the last chapter – it's a gem!). If you can swing both, even better! These are super handy, especially after a lengthy fast of 2 days or more, as they replenish vital electrolytes in your body.

Electrolytes, such as phosphate, drop faster as your body uses them to repair damaged cell parts when you resume eating. Maintaining the right balance of electrolytes is crucial because things can get a bit wonky after a prolonged fast. If they go off-kilter, you might experience something called refeeding syndrome, leading to symptoms like fatigue, weakness, irregular heartbeats, and more serious issues.

This occurs when you're not getting enough vitamins and minerals due to a habit of munching on too many processed and sugary foods or you have some health issues. So, take it slow and steady when breaking your fast – it's a safer bet!

- Do not catch up: Going all out with food right after fasting can undo the benefits of cutting calories during your fast. You might not see weight loss and could even gain some weight. Instead, take it slow and steady when breaking your fast!

C. Routine exercise

Keeping active is super important for staying healthy! Find an exercise you enjoy or can at least tolerate, and make it a regular thing. Exercise does a lot of good stuff for you – it lifts your mood, makes you stronger, and helps you limit the effect of your stress. The World Health Organization says doing sports at least five times a week for 30 minutes or three times a week for about 40 minutes is a great idea.

Here are the awesome perks of exercise: Moving your body isn't just a workout for muscles; it's a brain-boosting, memory-enhancing secret weapon against aging! Staying active keeps your brain young and your mind super smart.

And did you know your gut loves a good workout, too? Just like you hit the gym for muscles, your gut benefits when you get moving. It's like a party for the friendly bacteria—they multiply and thrive! As these buddies multiply, they work wonders for your immune system, helping you fend off germs and illnesses.

Want to keep that cholesterol in check? Dive into the world of quick and intense exercises with High-Intensity Interval Training (HIIT)! Whether it's sprinting, swimming, or cycling like the wind, or even just a brisk walk, the key is to push yourself, then ease back, and repeat as much as you can. Spice it up with moves like squats, push-ups, mountain climbers, plank, and burpees - the perfect recipe for a routine that tones and heals your body. And remember to wrap it all up with some nice stretching to keep your body feeling flexible and refreshed.

Additionally, when you get your body moving for more than an hour, autophagy happens in your muscles, making them feel all fresh and brand new, just like when you fast. You know those athletes who always seem to look so youthful? It's because their intense training sparks autophagy. But the good news is you don't need to be a pro athlete. Just an hour of fun activities like dancing, jumping rope, brisk walking, or swimming can do the trick.

While you're enjoying your physical activities, it's important to recognize the dangers of prolonged sitting, often called 'Sitting Disease' or a 'sedentary lifestyle.' Even if you exercise regularly, too much sitting can still harm your health. To combat this, make it a habit to stand up, stretch, and move around every thirty minutes. Simple changes, like standing during phone calls or walking to a colleague's office instead of sending emails, can make a big difference in your overall well-being.

D. Be the Expert in charge of your health and well-being.

"Taking care of yourself is the most powerful way to begin to take care of others"
Bryant H. McGill

1. Take Charge of Your Physical Health

Imagine you're on a journey to better health, and along the way, you have all these amazing guides like doctors, nutritionists, fitness coaches, and health experts. They're like your trusty companions, offering advice, tools, and even medications to help you navigate.

However, the truth remains: you're in charge here. You get to choose the direction of your health journey. If you're sick, it's up to you to see a doctor. Taking medication is your call. Likewise, deciding to fast based on a nutritionist's advice is also on you. While these experts offer helpful guidance, ultimately, you have the power to make decisions that lead to a healthier and happier life.

So, when it comes to taking control of your health, it's mostly about not letting excuses steer your decisions. Its also understanding and getting good at listening to what your body is telling you.

Ditch Excuses

Do you ever find yourself saying things like, "I eat because I don't want to waste food," or "I don't eat the way I should because my partner isn't supportive," or "I'm too busy with work to exercise"? It's common to make excuses like these, but let's face the truth: none of us are irreplaceable.

Think about it: if something were to happen to you, your office and your partner might miss you for a while, share some heartfelt stories, but eventually, they'd move on. It's tough to accept, but it's true. So, the next time you convince yourself that work is an obstacle to your commitment to exercise, remember that you control your priorities and can adjust them. And when you're tempted to finish off your kid's plate just to avoid wasting food, remember there are other options. You can store leftovers in the fridge or leave them out for the next meal.

Making excuses won't help you shed those extra pounds, tone your thighs and arms, boost your energy, ease food discomfort, or heal. Instead, they will only get in the way of your journey to wellness.

Learn to Communicate with Your Body

Its all about building a strong and mutually beneficial connection with your body. Think of your body as this incredible machine that's always sending you messages to keep everything running smoothly. All you have to do is tune in and listen to your body. Pay attention to how you feel and how your body responds to your diet and lifestyle. Then, take action to prevent and reverse disease. Your body's messages can be like cheers when you make healthy choices or protests if you don't respect its needs. It's up to you to tell the difference.

Your body protests in various ways. For example, you feel tired and uncomfortable when you overeat, right? But does it lead you to stop eating when your body signals it's full and content? As the captain of your health, it's your job to lay down your fork when you're satisfied, even if there's still food on your plate. This helps you take back your power over food. I bet many of us struggle with this.

Also, if your belly gets bigger (check out tips to reduce belly fat in chapter 4), your body might be urging you to shed weight to stave off chronic conditions like type 2 diabetes, hypertension, cholesterol, and other heart diseases.

Feeling off after eating a certain food? maybe bloated? That's your body's way of saying, 'Hey, something's not right! Watch what you are eating!'. It could be that the food you ate isn't agreeing with you—maybe it wasn't cooked properly or it's not jiving with your digestion.

Ever wonder why you sometimes feel like eating more than usual? It could be because your body reacts to not getting enough sleep or being stressed for other reasons. This can throw off the balance of the hormones that control hunger and fullness, called ghrelin and leptin. By prioritizing good sleep, physical activity and relaxation, you can bring back balance and regulate your hunger levels. Understanding these cues helps you make better choices for a healthier life!

Ever wonder what your ideal food portion size is? The truth is, no scientific study or diet plan knows your needs better than you do. Food guidelines and studies are a good starting point, but your own mindfulness and intuitive understanding of yourself are more finely tuned and personalized. Finding your ideal food portion sizes is a gradual process of adjustments. Trust your inner wisdom and your body's signals for a healthier and more satisfying approach to meals. Remember that the boss of your health journey is… you!

I'd like to draw your attention to the habit of forcing yourself to eat when you're sick and not hungry. You were taught to believe it will "give you some strength." But have you ever considered that maybe your body is trying to tell you it needs a break from food? Eating requires digestion, which needs energy. When your body's defense system is battling illness, it needs to gather its resources to fight diseases more efficiently. So, when you are sick and not hungry, it might be because eating is a distraction that diverts your body's energy from the battle going on inside. If your sick body needs food, you'll feel hungry—unless you're unconscious.

On the flip side, when you treat your body well, it shows gratitude. Think about how great you feel after a good workout - those happy hormones flooding your system, lifting your mood and boosting your energy. Regular exercise keeps you fit and full of vitality. And when you enjoy a balanced meal, your body gets a steady supply of energy, keeping cravings and energy crashes at bay. Also, fasting work wonders, making you feel and look younger and more vibrant. These are all ways your body celebrates the five-star care you give it!

Medications are not always the solution.

Now, imagine food as your body's natural medicine, echoing the wisdom of Hippocrates, one of the fathers of medicine. While doctors might prescribe quick-fix and long-term pills for ailments, making changes in what you eat and how you live can address the root causes. For example, a painkiller might take away your headache, but it doesn't fix what's actually causing it. This is similar to how medications like Metformin for blood sugar or statins for cholesterol work. Metformin can lower your glucose and improve insulin sensitivity, but it doesn't empower your body to handle these things on its own. So, you end up depending on it long-term because it doesn't address the root issue. It's like having a leaking ceiling—if you only dry the wet area and paint over the stains without fixing the leak, the problem persists, weakening the ceiling until it eventually cracks and falls. Until you address the source of the leak, you're just covering up the damage with more paint. This is similar to what these pills do to your health.

On the bright side, you can often tackle some health problems without meds by making simple tweaks to your diet and lifestyle. These changes can make a big difference and help you avoid side effects from pills, like low testosterone, erectile dysfunction, or sleep issues that can come with medications such as statins.

2. Take Charge of Your Mental Health

You know how important it is to take care of your body to stay healthy. But let's be real here: staying physically fit is just one piece of the health puzzle. Your mental well-being, though less visible, holds incredible sway over your life. How can you achieve happiness with a great body if your self-esteem is low? The fact is, even if you're in great physical shape, you won't truly enjoy life if your mental well-being isn't in check.

Just like you prioritize your physical health with daily exercise and nutritious food, it's essential to give your mind the same attention and care it needs to stay healthy. Striving to become the best version of yourself, both physically and mentally, can lead to genuine happiness.

In the previous chapters, I discussed physical health through stuff like eating traditional food, taking breaks from eating, and moving your body to keep it healthy. Now, let's explore how you can ensure your mind stay happy and healthy, too!

Mind's wellbeing

Our mind is like the invisible part of us that often gets ignored. When our mind struggle with issues like eating disorders, self-sabotage, low self-esteem, sadness, depression, anxiety, or anger management difficulties, we tend to attribute it to a mysterious plot orchestrated by a jealous neighbor or relative. It's common to search for external explanations for internal struggles. We don't usually talk openly about our feelings, and don't promote healthy ways to manage them. We still judge and shame some feelings as "bad," so people only share what they think is acceptable. People hide the "bad" feelings like humiliation, rejection, abandonment, betrayal, or depression.

But keeping these feelings secret doesn't make them disappear. They quietly grow inside us and affect everything we do. They hide under the feeling of not being good enough or the tendency to blame others for our problems because we struggle to take responsibility for our actions. They also manifest in how we rely too heavily on others for support because we're afraid to try on our own. This pattern of behavior prevents us from dealing with our problems in a healthy way.

Have you ever wonder why some overweight folks can't commit to a diet or exercise routine even though they really want to get back in shape? Losing weight or committing to a healthy lifestyle isn't just about knowing what to eat and how to exercise; it also needs motivation to take action, which comes from loving and caring for ourselves, all connected to our mental health.

Here are some tips to nourish the mind and make it an ally, not an enemy:

Be Your Priority

Improving yourself starts with a bit of self-focus, and looking out for your own well-being. Trying to please everyone and tackle every problem around you can turn you into a stressed-out and controlling individual. And guess who feels the impact the most besides you? The people closest to you, like your kids, partners, and immediate family and friends. So, When you put yourself first and take care of your own needs, you're boosting your own happiness and your ability to care for your loved ones.

For example, when you're feeling low or stressed, don't you tend to be more irritable and impatient with your family and friends? Conversely, when you're feeling good, you're much more understanding and loving, right? This means taking care of yourself sets the stage for you to be the best version of yourself for your family.

 I bet you're familiar with airplane safety demonstrations. They always instruct parents to secure their own oxygen masks before assisting their children. This message cannot be clearer. if you're not in a good place yourself, you'll struggle to provide effective help. In fact, you might even add confusion to the mix.

Now imagine you're invited to dinner, but you're fasting. You might feel obligated to say yes to please your host, but deep down, you know it's important to prioritize your own needs. Would you decline or please the host? Remember, putting yourself first feels great. It spreads to those around you like a happy contagion.

Stress Relief: Boost Your Vagus Nerve with Breathing Techniques, Foot Massage, and more

You've learned how to handle stress by taking care of your body. Now, let's shift your focus to reducing stress by taking care of your mind.

Your body is no stranger to stress—whether it's from work, family, or daily life. When stressed, your body kicks into high gear: your heart races, blood pressure shoots up, and your senses become super sharp. This reaction is meant to help you deal with tough situations and find quick solutions to escape the threat. However, it's only meant to happen occasionally.

Trouble starts when you turn everyday challenges into constant threats, keeping your body in stress mode that produces too much cortisol. This stress hormone causes inflammation, heart trouble, type 2 diabetes, and other health problems in the long run.

Inside your body, there's something truly amazing called the vagus nerve. It starts in your brain, travels down your neck and throat, and then keeps going into your chest and abdomen. Along the way, it helps you swallow and speak, keeps your heart rate and breathing in check, and cares for your gut health and immune system. It even plays a role in reducing inflammation and controlling hunger and fullness—talk about a multitasker! But for now, let's focus on its stress relief power. The vagus nerve acts like a firefighter, calming things down after stress. It also helps balance your inner Yin and Yang, the opposite energies in Chinese culture, where Yang is linked to stress and action, and Yin to relaxation and restoration.

The exciting part about this fantastic nerve is that it just needs a little nudge to do its thing. By stimulating it, you can help your organs work smoothly and reduce your risks of getting sick from stress, as mentioned in the lifestyle drama triangle above. Now, you might be thinking, "How can I activate this nerve?" Well, it's as simple as daily meditation, breathing exercises, a good laugh, prayer, or foot massage. These activities can wake up the vagus nerve and help you find inner peace again.

There are some great breathing techniques that can really help you relax, boost your focus, and increase your oxygen levels by stimulating the vagus nerve.

One of these breathing techniques is Belly Breathing, also known as diaphragmatic breathing. It's great for handling short-term stress caused by things like arguments, tight deadlines, or unexpected events. In this breathing technique, you keep your chest still and let your belly rise as you inhale deeply, filling your lower lungs with air. When you exhale, your belly falls as the air leaves your lungs. In this exercise, it is important that your chest stays still while only your belly moves. It's all about deepening your breath to get more oxygen in.

Another awesome technique is Box Breathing. It's perfect for calming your mind. It is especially useful for people in high-stress jobs (military, athletes during competitions, etc.) or any other situations where you need to stay cool under pressure. This technique is super simple and works in four equal parts:

1. Breathe in slowly and deeply through your nose for a count of four seconds;
2. Hold your breath for a count of four seconds;
3. Slowly breathe out through your mouth for a count of four seconds;
4. Hold your breath again for a count of four seconds.

My personal favorite is Toning. It's fantastic for chronic stress such as work-related pressure, and persistent anxiety; and for emotional stress such as relationship issues, grief, or feelings of overwhelm. This technique involves making a steady vocal sound, like "Aaaaah" or "Oooooh," while you exhale. It might feel a bit weird, like an incantation, but the vibrations from the sound stimulate the vagus nerve and help you relax.

Here's how to do it:

1. Find a comfy spot;
2. Take a deep breath through your nose;
3. As you exhale, make a continuous, even sound that resonates in your body.

Practice any of these techniques for a few minutes and see how they work for you! and don't forget to thank me later!

Laughter, meditation and prayers are also great ways to stimulate your vagus nerve. Can you believe that just laughing can boost your vagus nerve and get those feel-good endorphins flowing? It's pretty amazing! Basically, having fun with friends or family and sharing a good laugh can lower cortisol, the stress hormone, making life's challenges a bit easier. Similarly Daily meditation and prayers are like a mini-vacation for your mind, helping you unwind and achieve a sense of calm and emotional balance.

Feet massages are incredibly relaxing. Your feet are like a map of your body, and hitting certain spots can give your vagus nerve a boost, making it easier to chill out and shake off stress. When you massage your feet, you trigger those feel-good hormones that help you relax, sleep better, and even ease migraines. So whether it's your partner pampering you or a session with an acupressure therapist, a foot massage is a fantastic way to tackle stress and feel great overall.

Dive Into Healing: Experience the Magic of Nature's Bathing!

Nature is like free medicine for your mind and body. Imagine taking a stroll on the beach or walking through a forest—it's like getting a dose of nature's healing power!

At the beach, you can feel the soft sand under your feet and enjoy the sea breeze. The air there contains iodine, salt, and magnesium, which are natural healers. In the forest, trees release anti-anxiety chemicals called terpenes into the air as you walk around.

These natural goodies are like boosters for your body and mind. Breathing in sea or forest air, or letting your skin soak up nutrients and sunlight, gives you a healthy dose of vitamins and therapeutic chemicals. They support your respiratory system, reduce stress, and make you feel happier.

Practice Gratitude

Have you ever realized how problems can take over? They become our entire world, and we forget all the awesome stuff around us.

I like to think of life as the vast universe containing a whopping two trillion galaxies. When we face a challenge, it is like a single galaxy going wrong. But Sometimes, we focus so much on this faulty galaxy that it becomes our universe. It overshadows the beauty of everything else in our universe—a universe filled with jobs, a house, our parents' being alive, our children, our health, our faithful friends, a loving family, and our ability to breathe, walk, see, smell, feel, touch, speak, and hear, etc. These everyday wonders often slip by unnoticed.

Do you remember when you last expressed love to your parents, partner, relatives, or friends? Do they know you care? Have you ever paused to appreciate how nature can display vibrant colors in summer and snowy white in winter, showing its incredible versatility? Our focus tends to fixate on challenges that represent just a tiny, temporary fragment of our existence.

So, are we being fair to ourselves? Gratitude steps in as a gentle reminder to appreciate this beauty and express thanks for it. Whether you're a creative artist, a skilled speaker, an entrepreneur, a great listener, handy with tools, or a captivating storyteller, gratitude unveils the power within you. Take a moment to list and appreciate your achievements and all that surrounds you. It prevents you from taking things for granted and helps you see the beauty in just being you. Gratitude encourages you to acknowledge and value the two trillion amazing galaxies of your universe, emphasizing the undeniable awesomeness of your life.

Taking care of yourself is a powerful gift for your body and mind. You deserve to put yourself first, get the right info, and make choices that keep you healthy and smart.

Susan:

the SET-FREE method has been pivotal in transforming my relationship with food. It has created a valuable space for me to make mindful choices and eat with consciousness. On top of that, fasting has boosted my endurance and resilience, giving me not just a leaner physique but also a significant improvement in my overall well-being.

Blessing:

Since I started 16-8 intermittent fasting, my energy levels have skyrocketed, and I now find it easier to fall asleep at night. My sleep quality has significantly improved, and I wake up feeling refreshed.

Chapter 4:

Health Hacks:
Conquer Disease and Own Wellness!

1. Why Tea is More Than Just a Drink

Teas are a fantastic addition to a healthy diet. Drinking them helps boost your body's defenses. Here are some of my favorites: honeybush, rooibos, moringa, green and black teas. Each one has its own set of antioxidants that complement each other. They're well-studied, popular, and easy to find in tropical countries.

Rooibos and Honeybush are sweet, caffeine-free herbal teas from South Africa. They're not just any tea – they're blends of leaves and stems with special powers. One cool thing they do is keep your blood sugar levels in check, making them great for fighting type 2 diabetes and belly fat.

These teas are packed with antioxidants like xanthones and flavanones, which help fight type 2 diabetes and protect your cells from cancer. They also tackle inflammation caused by belly fat and help with weight management. Plus, they're great for your heart and prostate health. And don't forget about green and black teas! They're antioxidant powerhouses too, working just as hard as Honeybush and Rooibos to keep you healthy.

In South Africa, people have long used honeybush tea to help with menopausal symptoms. This tea is packed with isoflavones and coumestan which are another set of powerful antioxidants. These antioxidants act like estrogen boosters, making menopause easier.

Last but not least, let's talk about the amazing moringa tea made from loose or powdered dry leaves. Unlike other teas, moringa leaves can be cooked like any other greens. Making tea out of them is just one of the many ways to tap into their incredible healing powers, which include heart protection, antidiabetic benefits, and anticancer properties. Thanks to its high protein, iron, and antioxidants content, moringa tea offers a host of health benefits, which you can find detailed in the "Vegetables and Fruits" section.

But remember, just sipping tea won't magically make you healthier. You need a plan. Teas work best when they're part of a healthy diet and lifestyle. They're best when you drink them without added sugar, but you can add flavors like lemon or cinnamon to make them taste even better.

2. Are Your Curves Healthy?

Before you start panicking about every inch of your body, let's get one thing straight – a little extra weight doesn't always equal being unhealthy. If it's spread out across your body, you're not on the fast track to chronic diseases. In some tropical corners of the world, having curves is even seen as a symbol of beauty. Just look at fabulous celebs like Yemi Alade, the Nigerian singing sensation; Omotola Jalade Ekeinde, the iconic Nigerian actress; Grace Decca, the Cameroonian star; and Samira Bawumia, the distinguished second lady of Ghana. Aren't they just stunning? The key is to keep an eye on that belly – it's like a health barometer. As you celebrate your curves, remember also to stay on track with your health goals.

But, appearances can be deceiving. Just because someone looks slim doesn't guarantee they're healthy inside. Some folks might be battling insulin resistance and hiding a stash of visceral fat that could spell trouble. So, being slim doesn't always equal good health. Look around – you might spot a friend, family member, or acquaintance who seems slim but is wrestling with things like Type 2 Diabetes, or heart diseases. These folks are often described as having a "Thin on the Outside, Fat on the Inside" (TOFI) condition. You may have noticed that some people in your family may not be fashion models but are healthier than many slim individuals.

Want to find out the best way to check your health risks? Let's discuss the commonly used Body Mass Index (BMI).

3. Is the BMI A Good Diagnostic Predictor?

The contradictions revealed in the previous section come from using Body Mass Index (BMI) as the main way to check body fat and assess risks for heart disease and Type 2 diabetes. BMI doesn't always give a clear picture of these health risks.

BMI, which is calculated from your weight and height, doesn't really measure your body fat accurately. It completely overlooks important factors like muscle mass and bone density. So, it ends up treating a fit athlete and someone with more body fat the same way, even though they're quite different inside.

In short, using BMI to gauge health risks is like trying to measure the ocean's depth with a teaspoon—it just doesn't work. As mentioned earlier, checking your belly size gives a clearer idea of your risk for chronic diseases.

4. Burn Your Belly Fat

Think of your body as an ever-changing adventure, just like life itself. It's not a smooth ride down a calm river; sometimes, it's more like a rollercoaster! You know those moments when everything feels a bit chaotic, like during puberty when you're growing and changing rapidly, or in adulthood when you might struggle with extra weight, especially after pregnancy. And let's not forget about menopause, a whole new journey for many. And guys aren't immune either with what's fondly known as a "beer belly."

What's the deal with these stubborn bellies? Well, Blame it on our crazy busy lives. Stress levels shoot up, pumping out cortisol like crazy, which in turn tells our bodies to produce more insulin, the hormone that stores fat. As a result, weight piles up around the middle.

Throw in a diet high in sugar, a couple of drinks here and there, and hormonal changes, and you've got the perfect recipe for growing bellies.

So, whether you're dealing with a menopause belly, a beer belly, or any other belly fat, it all boils down to one thing: your lifestyles are packing on the pounds in all the wrong places.

But no matter the cause, you can shrink that belly and get back in shape. First, let's understand more about menopause and beer bellies before I share some tips on how to lose belly fat effectively.

Get To Know Menaupose Belly

If you're a woman aged 45 or older going through perimenopause or menopause, you might find things getting a little tricky. Suddenly, your confidence might take a hit, especially when you notice extra weight creeping up around your belly. Your favorite clothes might not fit as nicely as they used to, making you doubt how you look, and feel less confident. You might even start questioning your worth. It's a tough time, both physically and mentally, and it's something we don't often discuss openly enough.

Well, the changes during menopause happen because of lower estrogen and progesterone levels. Estrogen helps control how your body uses energy (metabolism). It directly affects blood sugar and insulin levels. When estrogen drops, blood sugar and insulin levels rise, causing fat to collect in the belly, known as a "Menopause belly." This body change is exacerbated by the stress around this new life.

Now, when menopause throws hormones off balance, it also means waving goodbye to some muscle mass. The fewer muscles you have, the lazier your body becomes at burning calories, giving fat the green light to set up shop, especially in the arms and thighs – the spotlight areas for those unwelcome jiggles! This is where the wardrobe dilemma kicks in.

You opt for comfort over chic. And on scorching days, you might go the extra mile to cover up, sweating, just to feel incognito in your clothes.

Let's get real – navigating the twists and turns of this menopause journey is no joke. The struggles with the jiggles are undeniably real, and it's about time we started having open conversations about how to turn things around.

Get To Know Beer Belly

How about beer belly? It can happen to both men and women, especially when life gets busy with work, partners, and kids, and you relax with beer at home or social events. It might be time to reconsider that habit because many beers contain a sugar called maltose, made of two glucose molecules. So, drinking too much beer can actually grow that belly size!

Tips To Burn Belly Fat

The SET-FREE method is your ticket to keeping insulin low and shrinking that stubborn belly fat, whether it's a "Beer belly," "Menopause belly," or just plain old belly fat! Remember, the secret to long-term success is sticking with it and making small, steady changes that become habits you can keep up over time. So, begin with one or two tips and build on them as you move closer to your health goals. Here's is the SET-FREE plan:

- Start with fasting: Find a fasting routine that suits you. But remember, change it up every now and then to keep your body guessing. When you fast the same way all the time, your body can become less responsive. Fasting is super effective for trimming down that belly!

- Eat seasonal and traditional Foods: Stick to your usual, traditional foods and cooking methods—they're good for stabilizing insulin. It's okay to add sugar or fried or processed foods occasionally, but keep them as occasional treats.

- Reduce beer consumption: Drinking beer and alcohol in excess is also fattening, especially around the waist. Ethanol from beer and other alcohol tends to metabolize in the brain and liver, making bad fat that will go to your visceral and make you fat and sick.

- Manage your stress: Now, I'm not suggesting that some people can't handle stress like champs. In fact, a bit of stress now and then can be quite invigorating. But let's get real for a moment. Chronic stress has become the norm in our everyday lives. Regular physical activity, prayer, and meditation are fantastic ways to calm our mind and body. And don't forget about foot massages—they're like a magic trick for relaxation, letting go, and feeling fabulous!

- Take charge of your health: This means putting yourself first and giving your health the five-star treatment it deserves. It's time to kick those excuses to the curb!

- Hydrate with healing teas: Staying hydrated isn't just about quenching your thirst—it's also a hidden trick for fighting belly fat! Along with plain water, try those tropical teas I mentioned earlier. They're great companions on this journey.

5. How Can You Prevent and Treat Uterine Fibroids?

This is a big deal, especially for black women. Uterine fibroids are non-cancerous lumps that can cause heavy periods, anemia, infertility, and miscarriages. I'm sure many of you are currently dealing with or know someone struggling with fibroids. It almost seems inevitable. The truth is, we don't know exactly what causes them, but we do know that black women are more often affected. While some risk factors, like genetics, family history, and age, can't be changed, things like diet and lifestyle can be improved to make a difference in your life.

Fibroids are mainly linked to too much estrogen in the body that isn't being properly eliminated. Guess what's behind this? Belly fat and high insulin levels! Belly fat produces estrogen, and on top of that, Insulin increases inflammation, which stimulates an enzyme that produces even more estrogen. Fibroids thrive on estrogen, so the more estrogen in the body, the larger the fibroids grow and the worse the symptoms become.

Nutrition and Lifestyle Treatment:

Getting rid of excess estrogen is key for managing fibroids. It all starts with your gut. Frequent constipation, for example, can make it harder for your body to get rid of extra estrogen. So, eating traditional foods, and cutting down on inflammatory foods like processed food and sugar, will help your gut work better and eliminate excess estrogen properly.

Here are some SET-FREE tips to prevent and treat fibroids without relying only on surgery which does not treat the root cause.

1. Reduce Belly Fat: Burning belly fat (check out section 4 above for tips) reduces the sources of estrogen production which are mainly belly fat, insulin, and inflammation.

2. Reduce Inflammation: Eat mainly traditional food. Cut down on processed food, fast food, sugar and limit exposure to pollution to reduce inflammation.

3. Improve Gut Health: Take care of your gut by eating more fermented foods and fiber-rich foods like tubers, beans, peas, grains, and lots of vegetables. This boosts your gut health, reduces inflammation, and helps your body eliminate excess estrogen and other toxins.

By making these changes to your diet and lifestyle, you can help prevent fibroids and gradually bring your body back to a normal hormonal balance.

6. Reverse Type 2 Diabetes, High Cholesterol, and Hypertension: It's Possible!

"T2D is a curable disease, but as a dietary disease, it demands
a dietary treatment,"

Dr Jason Fung

"Stop using medicine to treat food,"

Dr. Sarah Hallberg

Years ago, when my mom faced challenges with type 2 diabetes and its issues, I felt helpless and couldn't do much to help her. We followed doctors' advice of a low-fat, low-calorie diet and more exercise, but it didn't save her. Back then, experts said type 2 diabetes was a chronic disease with complications as part of the normal progression. After my mom passed away in 2009, I changed my economics career to become a functional nutritionist.

I was keen on understanding Type 2 diabetes and cardiovascular diseases and finding ways to combat it. While pursuing my master's degree in nutrition, I discovered that my education was more geared towards preventing and managing these chronic diseases rather than reversing them. In the same line, my thesis focused on preventing Type 2 diabetes in Cameroon through dietary and lifestyle changes. While my years of practice were satisfying in some ways, it wasn't quite what I had envisioned. My real goal has always been to prevent and reverse diabetes. Feeling frustrated, I decided to take a break and dive into scientific research, exploring both conventional and alternative medicine, along with traditional methods, to expand my knowledge.

During my break, I got to know many healthcare professionals who questioned the old ways of doing things in medicine. They weren't satisfied with giving medicine to treat symptoms; they wanted to find different and better solutions, just like me. They were passionate about giving better care for chronic diseases like obesity, Type 2 diabetes, and heart problems. Each had to rethink how they practiced medicine because they needed more skills. It doesn't mean what they did before was wrong; it just means there's always more to learn!

These doctors went beyond their standard education and typical medical practices. They delved into the fundamentals of health—diet and lifestyle—to uncover the root causes of various health issues. They looked into many scientific studies about food that people didn't pay much attention to. What they found out is that a lot of illnesses, like Type 2 Diabetes and heart diseases, are strongly connected to what and how we eat. So, to reverse them, we need to change our diet and lifestyle, which is going back to the root cause. Medicine can only help control chronic diseases; it doesn't cure them.

They were intrigued by fascinating findings, such as the body's ability to heal through autophagy. These doctors unearthed underutilized information, and with that knowledge, they developed dietary strategies aimed at treating and even reversing diseases by altering our eating habits and lifestyles. They also recognize the value of medicine when necessary.

Hippocrates, the father of medicine, once said, "Let food be thy medicine and medicine be thy food." This really inspired these doctors to embrace this concept wholeheartedly. They use fasting as a powerful way to help the whole body regain balance, especially when dealing with long-term health issues. They also stress the importance of keeping our gut healthy because it plays a big role in preventing and treating diseases like obesity, high blood pressure, heart disease, and type 2 diabetes. So, what could be better for our gut health than sticking to traditional foods?

More and more doctors are shifting the approach to managing heart disease and Type 2 diabetes by focusing on diet as a primary treatment. This strategy, which is gaining popularity among healthcare professionals, emphasizes intermittent fasting, quality carbs, and healthy fats—based on the proven benefits of good fats that I covered earlier.

Intermittent fasting becomes like a super-medication for those dealing with chronic diseases. Just like you wouldn't skip your prescribed meds when you're on the road to good health, you shouldn't skip out on this dietary plan either. Stick to the guidelines, stay on track, and be a champ with your discipline – that's the key to seeing the best results and beating your disease.

One prominent figure in this movement is **Dr. Jason Fung,** a Canadian nephrologist and a globally recognized expert on intermittent fasting. Renowned for his insightful books, such as "The Obesity Code: Unlocking the Secret of Weight Loss," "The Diabetes Code: Prevent and Reverse Type 2 Diabetes Naturally," and "The Complete Guide to Fasting," Dr. Jason Fung has pioneered a significant shift in the management of Type 2 Diabetes. Transforming type 2 diabetes from a progressive and degenerative disease to a potentially reversible one, he has successfully treated thousands of prediabetes and type 2 diabetes patients through a combination of intermittent fasting and a low-carb diet. Dr. Jason has developed a comprehensive program, allowing individuals to naturally heal from type 2 diabetes by incorporating fasting into their lifestyle.

As we delve further into this transformative approach to managing chronic metabolic diseases, another notable figure in this movement is the late **Dr. Sarah Hallberg**, an American Osteopathic doctor. Dr. Hallberg has left an indelible mark by positively impacting the lives of numerous patients, guiding them to reclaim control over their health and completely reverse type-2 diabetes solely through dietary interventions.

Now, let's turn our attention to **Dr. Pradip Jamnadas**, an esteemed American medical professional. Serving as the founder and medical director of Cardiovascular Interventions for over 31 years in Central Florida, Dr. Jamnadas is widely recognized for his expertise in interventional cardiology. Awarded Orlando Top Doctor by Orlando Magazine for over a decade, Dr. Jamnadas has consistently demonstrated exceptional skills in his field.

What sets Dr. Jamnadas apart is his innovative use of fasting as the primary line of treatment for his patients dealing with Type 2 Diabetes and Cardiovascular Disease. With over a decade of successful implementation, Dr. Jamnadas has integrated fasting into his medical practice, showcasing its effectiveness in addressing these chronic conditions. To learn more about Dr. Pradip Jamnadas and his approach, visit his website at https://orlandocvi.com/medical-providers/dr-jamnadas/.

Shifting our focus to India, we encounter **Dr. Roshani Sanghani,** a specialist in Endocrinology, Diabetes, and Metabolism. Dr. Sanghani is particularly dedicated to addressing hormone imbalances in her patients. Through tailored diet and lifestyle changes, she empowers individuals to achieve optimal hormone balance, promoting better health while reducing dependency on medication. Having aided thousands dealing with weight-related diseases, including type 2 diabetes patients, Dr. Sanghani has facilitated significant improvements and even reversals. To delve deeper into her work, you can explore her contributions on her website at https://reisaanhealth.com/.

Lastly, we turn our attention to **Professor Robert H. Lustig**, an American neuroendocrinologist at the University of California. A prominent advocate against the harmful effects of sugar, Prof. Lustig has delved into the nuanced impact of different sugar types on our health and weight. Renowned for his best-selling books such as "Fat Chance: Beating the Odds Against Sugar, Processed Food, Obesity, and Disease," and the widely-viewed video "The Bitter Truth" recorded in 2009, Prof. Lustig continues to contribute significantly to the discourse on nutrition and health. You can explore his website at https://robertlustig.com/ for further insights into his work.

In my new journey to tackle chronic diseases, I team up with doctors to help patients with Type 2 Diabetes and cardiovascular diseases, just like functional nutritionists do. While I guide people on diet and lifestyle, doctors monitor diabetes medications. For example, intermittent fasting and medications like metformin both help lower blood sugar. However, using them together can be a powerful combo that might lower blood sugar too much. Regular doctor visits ensure your medication doses are just right and that your health is closely monitored. Your doctor will gradually reduce your medication until you might no longer need it. This also works for patients dealing with issues like hypertension, high cholesterol, and other heart diseases. It's important to have your doctor and nutritionist on board as you try to reverse heart disease and type 2 Diabetes through fasting, diet, and lifestyle changes.

7. Keep Your Prostate Healthy

The prostate is a multitasking organ typically about the size of an African bitter kola. It helps make and store the fluid that nourishes and moves sperm, and it's also involved in peeing.

Once you hit around 50, keeping your prostate healthy becomes a big deal. Suddenly, the worry about prostate cancer becomes real. On top of that, the prostate tends to grow as you age. Scientists aren't totally sure why, but things like not getting enough exercise, carrying extra weight around your middle, and just the natural changes of aging all play a part.

Now, the good news is having a bigger prostate doesn't mean you're more likely to get cancer. Phew!

However, If you notice signs like feeling like you haven't emptied your bladder, a weak pee stream, a sudden urge to pee, trouble controlling your pee, or needing to pee a lot, it's time to pay attention. The smart move? See a doctor. They can do some checks to figure out what's going on. Even though a bigger prostate itself might not be life-threatening, it can mess with your daily routine if things get complicated.

So, at 50 and beyond, your prostate needs some extra care, whether you're noticing symptoms or not. Taking care of it now can make a big difference in your health. Check out these simple diet and lifestyle tweaks to keep your prostate in top shape. Not only can they help with symptoms like prostate enlargement, but they can also significantly lower your risk of prostate cancer.

Keep fit and sexually active: First off, let's talk about being active. Moving around and exercising regularly helps keep your prostate in good shape. So, make sure you're getting some exercise – it's like a weapon against prostate issues. Also, the more you are sexually active, the more you decrease your risk of prostate cancer. The simple process of ejaculation is enough to help keep the prostate healthy, so if you're flying solo, no worries—you've got it covered!

Tidy up your lifestyle: Do you find yourself reaching for alcohol multiple times a week? Or maybe you're a smoker? It's important to know that your prostate, a carcinogen-sensitive organ, can be influenced by these substances and increase your risk of cancer. Cutting back on alcohol or cigarettes, or even better, saying goodbye to them altogether, can really benefit your prostate health.

Reduce your belly fat: Now, the villains we need to tackle are obesity and belly fat. They are a real threat to your prostate. Obesity and, especially, belly fat are like the bad guys, causing all sorts of health troubles, including problems messing with your prostate health. But don't worry, I've got some tricks to help you lose that belly fat. Check out section 4.4 for the deets.

Watch what you drink: Alongside your regular water intake, I highly recommend teas, whose benefits I discussed earlier. Now, let's chat about coffee! Sip on some unsweetened coffee every day—it's like a shield for your prostate, keeping it healthy and lowering the risk of things like prostate cancer. If you've got heart concerns, though, it's wise to chat with your doctor before diving into coffee.

Hold on to your bedtime beverages because what you sip before hitting the hay can impact more than just your dreams! Too many bathroom trips disrupt your beauty sleep and throw a party in your health lane. We all know the value of beauty sleep—it's like a power-up that keeps your heart and other organs in tip-top shape.

Specific protective foods: It's time for some tasty weapons: lycopene-rich foods. These are like the bodyguards for your prostate. Hunt down tomatoes, apricots, guavas, and watermelons. And here's a pro tip—cooking tomatoes boosts their lycopene power! Even canned diced or whole tomatoes can be just as effective, and sometimes even better!

Zinc is like a guardian for your prostate, keeping it strong and healthy. To load up on this mineral, munch on *Egusi* and try it out in different forms like *Egusi* sauce or *Egusi* pudding (also known as *Njuh, Nkono Ngond*, or *Nnam Ngon* in Cameroon). These dishes are like power-ups for your prostate.

But that's not all – you can also find Zinc in nuts, seeds, beans, lentils, chickpeas, and shellfish. Think of these foods as building a fortress around your prostate, making it extra tough and resilient. Don't forget your veggies – they're like the sidekicks that boost your immune system. Throw them in every meal, and you'll feel like the best version of yourself in no time.

Now, let's move on to the next topic: calorie counting! have you ever found yourself in a battle with your weight, staring down at your plate and wondering, "How many calories are hiding in here?" Maybe you've even turned to Google to investigate the calorie scoop before digging in. And oh, the worry—have you ever stressed about surpassing the daily recommended calorie limit? Have you wondered if your exercise routine can outsmart those sneaky calories you just ate? If you're nodding along, then I've got a topic that's totally up your alley!

8. Stop counting Calories to lose weight

How appealing is turning your meal into a math problem and figuring out the calories before taking a bite? Personally, it's not my thing. It feels like a mood killer during mealtime. And guess what? Some assumptions behind this whole calorie-counting idea aren't exactly true. Let me tell you why!

Assumption 1: You just need to exercise to lose weight. Untrue.

Let's discuss this myth about losing weight. Some people believe all you must do is exercise, but It's not that simple.

Imagine your body as a seesaw—on one side is what you eat, and on the other is how much you burn off through exercise. The idea is that if you eat something, you should burn it off with exercise, or it will turn into fat, and you will gain weight.

Now, check this out: say you gulp down a 600ml bottle of cola, packing in 248 calories and a whopping 16 teaspoons of sugar. Crazy, right? The recommended daily sugar amount is only about six teaspoons. Here's where it gets wild. You'd need to run about 7 km to burn off that cola. Who's up for that challenge? It's unrealistic for most of us. Plus, even if you somehow pull off that run, the energy boost from the cola is like a flash in the pan—quick but gone in a blink. You'd feel sleepy and tired and definitely not in the mood for a 7 km run. You can't just exercise away the effects of a not-so-healthy diet. It's like trying to run away from the consequences of a food choice. Sure, moderate exercise is good for your health, no doubt about it. But it doesn't work wonders when it comes to shedding those extra pounds. In fact, for many folks, working out might even make them hungrier, leading to more eating.

If we dream of major weight loss through exercise, here's the reality check. The usual recommendation is around 150 minutes a week or 30 minutes a day, five times a week. But to see significant weight loss, you'd have to kick it up a notch—think beyond the usual routine.

Imagine needing to exercise more intensely and more often than what's usually suggested. Sounds like a lot, right? Especially if you need to be training like those superathletes do for the Olympics. Achieving those significant weight loss goals would require some serious dedication—and let's be real, that's a story for very few of us.

Assumption 2: A calorie is a calorie. Untrue

Counting calories treats all foods equally; it does not dissociate nutritious food from empty calories (food containing many calories with few nutrients, like processed food and added sugars). It's like saying a plate of 100 calories of *Mandazi or Puff Puffs* is better for weight loss than 200 calories of *Dodo* greens or *Folon*, just because it's fewer calories. But that's not true!

Let's keep it real – does it sound right that 100 calories of *Babaqau* (a Fijian pancake) would be the same as 100 calories of coconut flesh? Not really, huh?

Your body is super smart. It doesn't see all calories as equals. So, saying "a calorie is a calorie" just doesn't cut it. Your body knows better! It's like it has a built-in calorie detective.

Your body knows how to handle natural, traditional foods—and it's no surprise they make your body happy! But processed foods and added sugars confuse your body. So, when it comes to calories, it's not just about how much you eat; it's also about what you eat. Quality matters!

That said, let's explore the main types of nutrients (fats, proteins, and carbs) that produce calories or energy as your body's fuel. Fat is the heavyweight champion, packing the most energy—nine calories per gram! Next is alcohol, which isn't a nutrient but delivers seven calories per gram. Then, we have protein and carbohydrates, delivering four calories per gram.

Here's where it gets interesting—even though fat has the most calories and the common belief is that it makes you gain weight, how can we then explain why the Keto diet, which is about 80% fats, 10% carbs, and 10% proteins, makes you lose weight? and a diet high in carbs, mainly processed ones and added sugars, is fattening?

So, your body has its rulebook for fat and sugar. They're treated differently, and understanding these nutrients is like having the keys to your body's energy kingdom!

Next time someone says, "A calorie is a calorie," you can tell them our body's team of hormones decides how things go down!

Assumption 3: your metabolism will remain constant. Untrue

So, when you try to eat fewer calories all the time, your clever body thinks, "Hmm, I need to save energy." It goes into survival mode, using less energy for everything—keeping your heart beating, keeping your body's temperature, organs doing their thing, and even growing muscles. This big energy-saving mode is called Resting Metabolic Rate (RMR), and it's about 60-80% of the energy you use. The higher your RMR, the faster you burn energy.

If you keep restricting calories, your RMR slows down, and it's like your metabolism is taking a little nap. As a result, your weight loss will also slow down.

Counting calories might seem like it's working at first, but soon, your weight loss hits a roadblock. Plus, this method can rob your body of important nutrients because it doesn't care much about your food quality. So, it's like a tricky shortcut that might not lead to the best results.

You've got the info now. As the boss of your health journey, it's your call to make the best decisions for you. You're in charge, Captain!

Irin :

I have been suffering thyroid issues and the SET-FREE method has greatly increased my energy level. Fasting has become a powerful ally in my journey towards better health, bringing a newfound vitality that I hadn't experienced before.

Chapter 5:

Healthy Kitchen Tips and Hacks

Remember, your health journey isn't about having a perfectly clean diet and lifestyle. It's more about finding the best balance for you. Here are some great tips on food combinations that can help you achieve that balance. Plus, I'll share some kitchen tool recommendations to help you smash that health goals.

1. Tips to Enjoy Added Sugars Occasionally

Here's a trick for an added sugar treat: pair it up with some food! If you're into sugary coffee, have it after a meal. Try sipping your sweetened *Bissap* or Ginger juice with seeds, nuts, *or Safu*. Also, when munching on bread, team it up with avocado, eggs, meat, butter, seeds, or nuts. This combo with fat, protein, and fiber will slow the sugar rush, reducing the insulin effect. Sweet, right?

2. Tips to Enjoy Grilled Meat and Fish With Less Health Damages

When you're grilling meat and fish, the fat and juice that drip into the fire create smoke filled with chemicals that can trigger inflammation and accelerate aging. This could potentially lead to long-term health issues. But hey, no need to stress! You can handle this cooking challenge like a boss. Before you start grilling, just trim off any extra fat and try this slick trick: marinate your meat for about 30min using lemon juice or vinegar to cut down on those nasty compounds. And remember to jazz up your grilled goodies with plenty of fresh veggies! Imagine pairing your juicy grilled meat or fish with some *Palusami* or sautéed leafy greens or even a mix of colorful sautéed veggies. Let's not overlook the delightful, zesty sauce perfectly matching your grilled fish and meat.

3. Tips on Choosing and Using Oils

Selecting Your Cooking Oil: Choosing the right oil is like selecting fresh, pest-free mangoes from the tree—it's about getting the nutritious and safe option. Quality is crucial! Consider this: Each oil has a smoking point, the temperature at which it starts misbehaving. Coconut, peanuts, red palm, and avocado oils boast high smoking points (177°C, 232 °C, 235°C, and 270°C), making them suitable for high-heat traditional cooking.

Now, let's talk about olive oil. Think of it as the delicate artist among oils—best suited for salads. If you intend to cook with it, opt for low heat and add it near the end. Each oil has unique superpowers, and the goal is to harness them for your health.

Choosing The Ideal Oil for Frying Food: Tropical oils should be your top picks if you enjoy deep or shallow frying. Nevertheless, it's always better to fry less for a healthier choice. So, take it easy on the frying adventures!

Reusing Frying Oil: When it comes to frying oil, don't make it a trilogy—using it more than three times can transform it into a sneaky villain known as trans fat. Trans fat messes with your cholesterol and blood pressure and poses serious risks to your heart and even other organs.

4. Tips for Cooling and Reheating Food

It's super important to keep your food safe when cooling and reheating. If your cooked food sits too long between 5°C (slightly chilled or damp) and 60°C (when tiny bubbles start to form as your food boils), it's like an open invitation for bacteria to come in and cause trouble. They can make you sick, from a simple upset stomach to more serious health issues. So, the plan is all about getting your food out of that danger zone fast. That means cooling and reheating need to happen quickly.

Cooling: When you're cooling leftovers, don't delay. Get that hot food into a cold water bath immediately, then pop it straight in the fridge. Keeping hot food in a fridge can increase its temperature, send it to the danger zone, and affect all the food there.

Reheating: When reheating, ensure the temperature is about 74°C (food simmering gently with more tiny bubbles). Slow reheating gives bacteria too much time to party and cause harm.

And if you know you won't eat your leftovers within the next 2 to 3 days, freezing them is a great option. It'll keep them fresh and tasty for months to come.

Blending Oils for Cooking: Sometimes, we need to be creative to get the combination of food we need. When it comes to oil, blending sesame oil (packed with omega-6) with flaxseed oil (high in omega-3) creates a powerful, winning team in your kitchen! This mix helps balance out the types of fats, making them friends instead of foes. It's all about reducing inflammation from omega-6 and maintaining a balanced ratio of omega-3 to omega-6 for better health.

5. Tips to enjoy traditional food using modern tools

Spending hours in the kitchen making traditional meals can be discouraging. The good news is that you've got some modern tricks in your back pocket now, so there's no need to stay in the kitchen for ages.

With some nifty kitchen gadgets, you can whip up those classic flavors in a flash. My teenager's a whiz at it—she's like a speedster in the kitchen! I learned tricks from her that made my life easier in the kitchen. So, go ahead, involve your children, blend old-school vibes with new-school flair, and get creative. Turn your kitchen into a fun playground with the following hacks!

Forget about struggling with grinding spices or grating coconut!

There are some tools that modern life has created to reduce cooking time. A mixer, for example. But suppose you don't have one, no worries! Just head to the local markets in tropical areas. They have manual or electric grinders that'll do the job without costing you an arm and a leg. These options are lifesavers. They can handle all sorts of dry or wet ingredients and even mix cassava leaves to get the same results as the pounded version! They grate coconut in the market and crush tough spices like *Ehuru*, *Pèbè*, and *Country onion*. Pre-made tropical spices are always available at local markets. African and Caribbean markets in Western countries are also great options.

Skip the Need for Tubers Pounding

Making *Achu*, a traditional Cameroonian dish, doesn't have to be an all-day affair like it was back in our grandparents' time. *Achu* consists of pounded cocoyam paired with a sauce made of red palm oil, spices, and meat. Thankfully, some awesome manual tools are available now that make the process a breeze, saving you loads of time. You can even use your blender to whip up some tasty yellow achu sauce in a snap! Craving *Mounou Mounouk*? A blender will blend the dates in no time.

Freezer Magic: Keeping Food Fresh

You can freeze your traditional food to keep it longer, especially when you live abroad. Greens, palm nuts, *Bobolo*, *Safu*, bushmeat, and tubers can all go in the freezer magic box. Pack them in sturdy plastic containers to keep most of the goodness intact—the flavors, colors, and taste! So, you can have a piece of home wherever you are.

Maximizing Quick Cooking Using a Pressure Pot

Another time-saving option is the pressure cooker. It makes cooking tough meats like cow legs and cow skin much quicker. It can save time for many other dishes.

6. Exploring Traditional Seasoning Tips and Options

Flavor enhancers like Maggi, Knorr, or Adjimoto have become staples in recipes, adding a delightful boost to the taste. These enhancers, available in cubes, liquids, and powders, contribute to the extra yumminess of your dishes. In my Jieumba language, we call these flavor boosters *kuitè Mban*, a small hard piece that makes food taste better. But these little things aren't the healthiest because they're highly processed and contain Monosodium Glutamate (MSG), which, at certain doses, is linked to some health issues. Can you remember how amazing our food tasted with traditional spices before these flavor boosters? So why do we all rush to those processed seasonings? Globalization, media, and aggressive marketing from the big food industry got us hooked! But it's not too late to rediscover and embrace those local spices.

Embracing Local Spices for Seasoning

Our grandparents totally rocked at using these spices, making their food naturally tastier with those enchanting seasonings. They deliver that sought-after umami flavor even better.

African dishes throw a spice party, bringing in hot flavors from peppers, ginger, and African pepper and pungent notes from *Country Onion*, *Alligator Pepper*, and *Uziza* seeds. Add the nutty touch of African nutmeg and the sweet and stringent twist from *Prekese* or *Tetrapleura*.

In the Caribbean and Pacific island's cuisine, spices dance to the unique blend of Indian and Asian cultures. Indian culture is dominant for a reason. In the late 1800s to early 1900s, as the large Indian community settled in the Pacific and Caribbean, they introduced a diverse array of spices. These spices offer a wide range of options to blend flavors, enhance the deliciousness of food, and promote healing. Some of these delights include curry, nigella, turmeric, garam masala, cardamom, cumin, mustard seeds. Additionally, coconut and its derivatives play a central role in the cuisine of these islands, featuring prominently in most dishes.

Creating Flavors With Homemade Broth

The broth is a blend of meaty bones and veggies that adds a subtle taste explosion to any dish. You can make broth from all sorts of bones—fish, shellfish, beef, lamb, chicken, you name it!. It is more than a standalone experience. Pour it into any savory dish that requires water, and voilà —you've elevated your meal's nutrition and flavor. Feeling adventurous? Take it a step further and savor it as a comforting soup. If you're eager to try your hand at making this nutritional elixir, the detailed recipe and health benefits await you in the dedicated next chapter!

Utilizing Dried Seafood for Seasoning

In tropical countries, there's a culinary secret weapon that turns ordinary meals into extraordinary meals—dried fish and crayfish. These tiny marvels elevate the taste of food to a whole new level, so much so that you might even consider ditching the salt!

These are a delightful combination of sweet and salty flavors that make every bite delicious. Sprinkle crayfish or add dried fish to almost anything – sauces, veggies, fried rice, greens, sautéed cocoyam, or dalo. When you combine them with raw palm oil or coconut oil in your cooking, it's like a burst of amazing flavors!

Believe me, it surpasses the magic of those stock cubes. If you're eager to transform your meals into a flavor-packed journey, this dynamic duo is the way to go!

Crafting Your Aromatic Seasonings

We've got stuff like *Benni* (see recipe in the next section), made from locust bean powder widely used in West African countries. There's also *Ogiri,* made from fermented sesame or Egusi paste. We toss these into sauces like okra or egusi to make the taste boom—that umami goodness!

Now, let's hop over to the Pacific and Carribean. Picture this – coconut milk, creamy curry, turmeric, fennel, and more. These flavors jazz up sauces, grains, and anything else.

7. Guidance and Suggestions for Cookware

Let's chat about a kitchen habit many of us picked up from our parents and communities—cooking in aluminum pots. Back home, these pots are the first choice. They're cheap, heat up super fast, and prevent burning. So, it's no surprise that almost every African family, even those living abroad, has a set of these shiny pots. We think they're unbeatable. However, what isn't well advertised is that aluminum pots leach particles into food during cooking, making us consume aluminum every day in our meals. Keep in mind that we already encounter aluminum from various sources, such as the air we breathe, aluminum foil used in cooking, and processed foods and drinks. Can you guess why table salt, sugar, and baking soda stay dry and pour easily? It's because of aluminum. It seems to be everywhere.

You've got to be a bit careful with it because when the level of aluminum in our body surpasses its limit, it can lead to problems affecting our kidneys, liver, breathing, and even our brain, potentially leading to issues like Alzheimer's.

There are alternatives pots that can meet your cooking needs with lower health risks than aluminum. Here are my picks.

Stainless steel: The top choice is stainless steel! These are the best cookware options, especially the high-quality ones. They're super safe—medical professionals even use top-notch stainless steel for everything from scalpels to prosthetic implants. So, it's definitely safe enough for your kitchen!

Coated cookware: Next up, coated cookware. The coating protects your food from sneaky metals. It is like a shield to keep the bad stuff out. But, if that coating gets a scratch, it's like a little hole in their shield, and metals like aluminum might try to get in your food. Coatings like copper, tin, and nickel can be a bit iffy, so if you're a fan of coated cookware, consider swapping them every 2 to 3 years – or even more often if you can swing it.

Choose wooden spoons to cook with: Wooden spoons are great because they don't get hot, making them safer and more comfortable for stirring hot foods. Plus, they're non-reactive, so they won't mess with the taste of acidic foods like tomato sauce or vinegar, keeping your dishes flavorful and healthy. They're also gentle on your pots, so no worries about scratches. Just remember to swap them out if they crack, to avoid any moisture that could lead to mold or bacteria. If you prefer silicone spoons, make sure to pick ones made from food-grade silicone, which is free from harmful chemicals like BPA and phthalates.

Choose parchment paper over aluminum foil and plastic wraps for steaming food: When banana leaves aren't available, we often turn to plastic or aluminum foil, which are both harmful. Cooking Moyi Moyi, Ivy, and Nguessan meleu with plastic releases toxic and cancer-causing compounds like BPA. A safer option is to wrap your food in parchment paper first, then add a layer of aluminum foil for secure protection without direct contact with your food.

Choose coolers over plastic wrap to keep food warm: Using cling film to wrap your hot *Foufou, Ugali, Posho, Nsima, or Akple* to keep them warm isn't the best option—you're still inviting harmful chemicals. If you don't have a cooler, why not go traditional? Wrap the food container with heavy clothes.

Cleaning kitchen utensils: Now, let's talk about cleaning your kitchen squad. Be gentle. Use a soft sponge or brush with the right cleaner – like stainless steel cleaner for stainless steel pots. If there's stubborn food stuck on, give your pot a cozy soak in hot water with baking soda for fifteen minutes. Did you get a burnt pot because you got caught up in this awesome book? No worries! Boil some water in it to loosen the burn. If it's still stubborn, give it a good scrape with a wooden spoon to help clean it up.

Chapter 6:

Tropical Traditional Recipes
and Global Inspirations

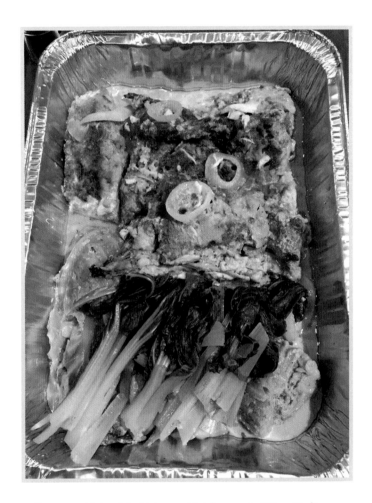

Coconut Fish with Chinese Cabbage: A Fijian Delicacy

Let's spice up our meals with a dash of creativity! Thanks to YouTube and social media, you don't need a passport to explore amazing recipes from around the world. Your local goodies can turn into global delights right in your kitchen. Get ready for a culinary adventure without leaving home!

1. Stock

Meat and fish stocks are widely used in traditional cuisines worldwide, touching every corner of the globe, including Tropical countries. These flavorful stocks aren't just limited to the kitchen; they've also made their mark in traditional medicines. I'm all about that stock life—it's the ingredient that brings almost all of my dishes to life.

A good stock, or bone broth, should have a magical quality—it jiggles and bounces when cooled, a sure sign that it's been crafted with care. Forget about those seasoning cubes with questionable ingredients! A well-made stock is the real deal, bursting with flavor without any need for additives like MSG found in seasoning cubes.

The amazing thing about stocks is that they are versatile. They make your food taste better, and are key players in sauces and many dishes. They also bring in extra nutrients, making your meal even healthier. And don't forget about the marrow at the end of a beef stock – it's perfect for spreading. It's like having the ultimate kitchen multitasker!

Health benefits of stock

Let's talk about the powerhouse of health benefits that come with these stocks! During the cooking process, a touch of acidity, like wine or vinegar, works its magic, coaxing essential minerals from bones, cartilage, marrows, and veggies and turning them into electrolytes. And guess what? Electrolytes are like the VIP pass for minerals in a form that our bodies easily digest and utilize. But that's not all – the protein-rich gelatin that emerges from these stocks isn't just good for texture; it's a digestive aid. Gelatin has been used to treat gut disorders and some chronic diseases. It's fantastic for your joints and makes your skin super healthy. It's like a cozy hug for your insides!

Now, here's a fun tidbit: in some African traditions, fish heads are believed to contribute to men's virility. Take Cameroon, for instance—the fish head is like a treasure for men; they absolutely love it! Rumor has it that adding special ingredients to it might just cast a love spell to bind your man even closer. Now, that's some flavorful folklore for you!

1.1. Fish Stock

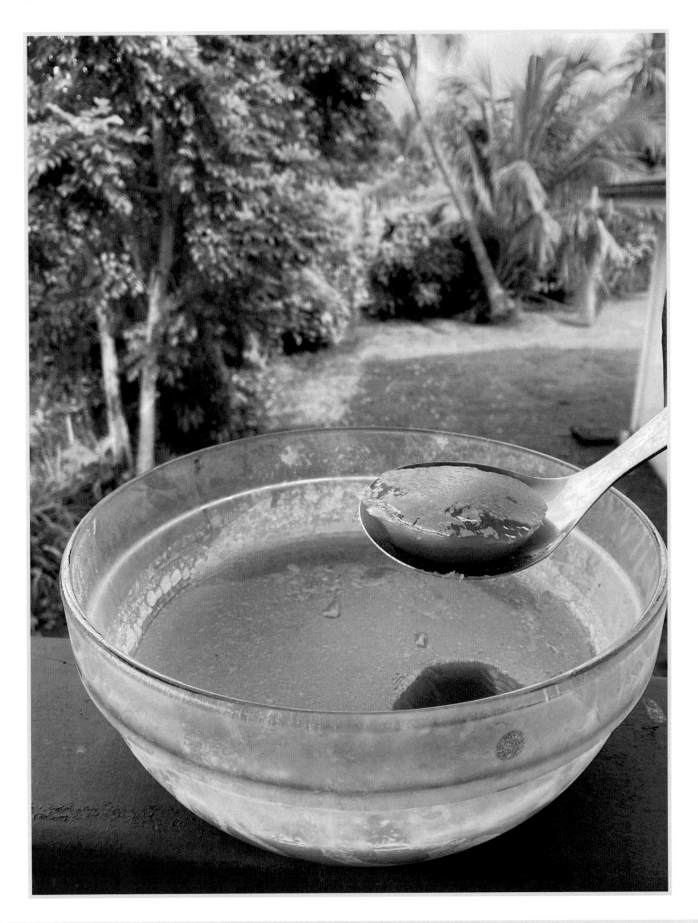

Ingredients

3 to 4 whole carcasses, including heads of non-oily fish such as sole, turbot, rockfish, or snapper
2 Tablespoon butter
2 onions coarsely chopped
1 carrot coarsely chopped
Several sprigs of fresh thyme
Several sprigs parsley
2 bay leaves
½ cup dry white wine
¼ cup vinegar
3 liters of cold filtered water

Process

Melt butter in a large stainless steel pot, then add the vegetables and cook gently for about 30 minutes until they're soft. Pour in the wine and bring to a boil. Add the fish carcasses and cover with cold, filtered water. Stir in the vinegar and bring the mixture to a boil, skimming off any scum and impurities that rise to the top. Tie the herbs together and add them to the pot. Reduce the heat, cover, and let it simmer for at least 4 hours, or up to 24 hours. Use tongs to remove the carcasses, then strain the liquid. Allow it to cool before transferring it to the fridge. Once chilled, remove any congealed fat, then package the stock into pint-sized containers or for the freezer to store long-term.

Credit: Nourishing Traditions Cookbook

1.2. Beef stock

You'll notice I use different types of bones for beef stock, and there's a good reason for that. Knuckles, bones, and feet provide most of the gelatin, while bone marrow adds nutrients like collagen and vitamin B12, plus extra flavor. Meaty bones, meanwhile, contribute color and additional taste.

Ingredients:

2kg beef marrow and knuckle bones
1 calve foot cut in pieces (optional)
1.5 kg meaty ribs or neck bones
4 liters or more cold filtered water
½ cup vinegar
3 onions coarsely chopped
3 celery sticks, coarsely chopped
Several sprigs of fresh thyme, tied together
1 teaspoon dried green peppercorns, crushed
1 bunch parsley

Process

Place the knuckle marrow bones, and calf food in a very large pot with vinegar and cover with water. Let stand for one hour. Meanwhile, in the oven, place the meaty bones in a roasting pan and brown at 160 degrees Celsius. When well browned, add to the pot along with the veggies. Pour the fat out of the roasting pan, add cold water, set over a high flame, and boil, stirring with a wooden spoon to loosen up coagulated juices. Add this liquid to the pot. Add additional water, if necessary, to cover the bones, but the liquid should come no higher than within 2.5 cm of the pot's rim, as the volume expands slightly during cooking. Bring to a boil. A large amount of scum will come to the top, which you should skim off with a spoon. Reduce the heat and add the thyme and crushed peppercorns.

Simmer for at least 12 hours and up to 72 hours. Just before finishing, add the parsley and simmer for another 10 minutes.

Remove the bones and strain the stock into a large bowl to get a deliciously nourishing and clear broth. Let it cool to room temperature, then refrigerate it to chill. Once chilled, remove the congealed fat and package the stock in a ziplock bag before freezing for long-term storage.

You can also make lamb stock using neck bones and riblets. I want to give a special mention to my Sahelian brothers and sisters here.

Credit: inspired by Nourishing Traditions cookbook

2. African Umami Mix Spices flavors

Ditch the processed stock cubes and go for traditional seasonings to get a mouthwatering umami kick. You'll find tastier and healthier options that deliver the flavor you're looking for. Once you experience the richness of these natural ingredients, you won't want to go back to commercial stock cubes. And hey, don't forget to thank me later!

James:

I had my share of challenges with intermittent fasting, battling frequent breaks in my routine, and dealing with weight fluctuations. But after hitting a plateau and facing health issues like elevated blood sugar and cholesterol, I decided to make a drastic change. I bid farewell to added sugars, processed carbs, and embraced a more structured fasting approach—adopting one meal a day and 48-hour fasts weekly.

The results were astounding. In just two weeks, I shed 5 kgs and felt a surge in energy levels. Fast forward three months and my medical checkup delivered some fantastic news – my cholesterol and blood sugar levels were back to normal. What's even more remarkable, a childhood allergy that used to plague me with constant sniffing seems to be a thing of the past. Intermittent fasting and the SET-FREE method not only transformed my physique but also brought unexpected health improvements.

2.1. Benny

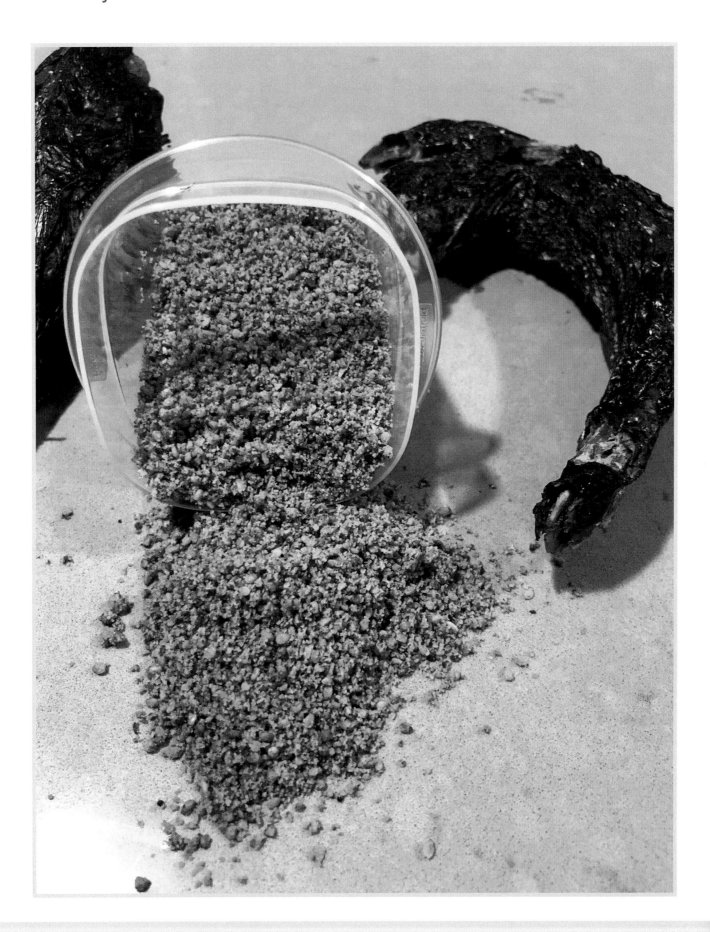

Craving that authentic African Umami taste? Look no further—*Benny's* got your back! You can sprinkle it as a condiment on your greens, like cassava and potato leaves, pair it with rice, or go all out and enjoy it with boiled cassava, sweet potatoes, yam, or cocoyam.

I stumbled upon *Benny* a few years ago at a friend's house, and let me tell you, I got hooked real quick. Now that I know how to cook it, you'll always find it hanging out in my kitchen closet, ready to bring that burst of flavor.I don't just enjoy it with meals; sometimes, I eat it alone because it's just that good!

Health benefits

The main star, sesame, is loaded with fibers. That means it's fantastic for digestion and reduces the risk of obesity and chronic diseases. The healthy fat content is like a shield against high cholesterol, promoting heart health. And don't overlook the pepper – it's boosting your digestive fluid production, making digestion a breeze. *Benny's* a health party on your plate!

Ingredients

½ kg Sesame seeds
2-3 tablespoons Cayenne pepper or as you wish
2 Bonga (popular dried fish in West and Central Africa) or other fish like sardine.
Piece it and remove all bones.
Salt

Process

In a stainless steel pot, roast sesame seeds until they become brown. Stir constantly so that they don't burn. Let them cool, and add pepper, salt, and *Bonga* to the seeds. Grind all these dry ingredients into a blender. Your *Benny* is ready! That's the African Umami taste we are talking about!

You can enjoy it with boiled cassava, cocoyam, or sweet potatoes. You can also use it as a condiment and add it to your greens, such as cassava and potato eaves, o enjoy it with rice.

2.2. Ogiri

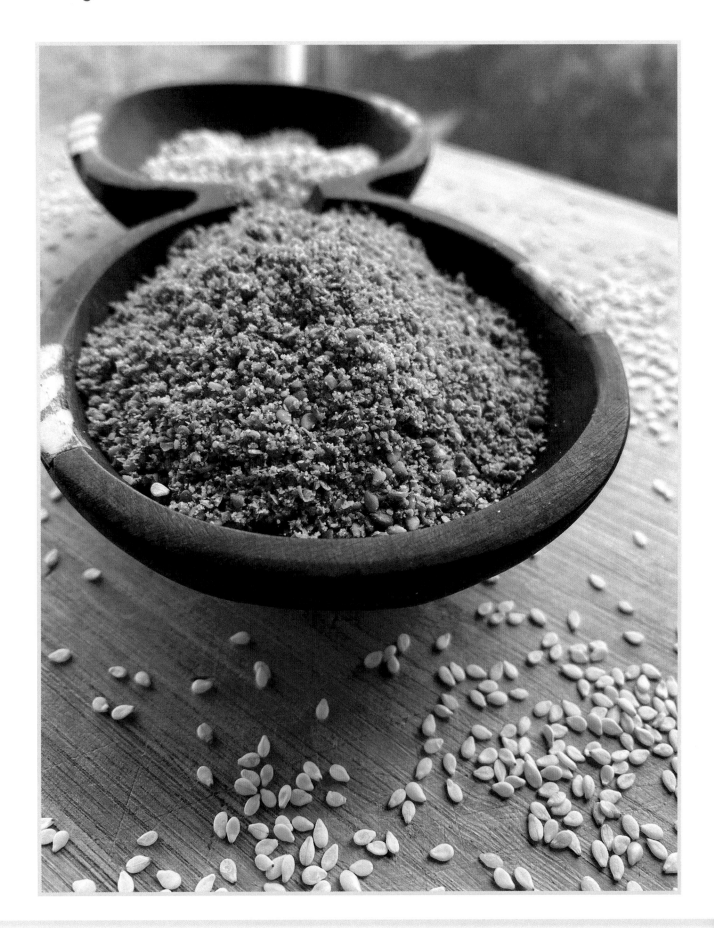

Have you ever heard of *Ogiri*? It's a traditional West African condiment from fermented seeds like sesame or egusi. It has a robust smell, like cheese or *Bobolo*. You'll find it stealing the culinary spotlight among the Yoruba and Igbo folks in Nigeria and the Sierra Leonese.

But what's the magic? *Ogiri* gives your food that unmistakable African Umami taste. Picture it as a flavor that can level up your stew, okra, or any veggie sauce with its unique aroma.

Health benefits

Ogiri is a probiotic powerhouse, thanks to its fermentation process. It brings some gut-friendly goodness along with it!

Ingredients

3 cups white sesame seeds
1 and a half cups water. Water must cover the sesame seeds.
Banana leaves to wrap *Ogiri* for roasting.
You can substitute banana leaves with parchment paper.

Process

Pour the sesame into a glass container and cover with water. Keep it at room temperature with the lid on for about nine days. Then, to further boost the flavor, you can wrap small portions of it in banana leaves and bake at 105 degrees Celsius for 3 to 4 hours. Your *Ogiri* is ready! Keep it in a well-sealed container. It stores for up to months in a dry place. If you live in a humid environment, you should store it in the freezer.

Note: You can substitute with parchment paper if you don't have banana leaves.

2.3. Fermented African locus bean.

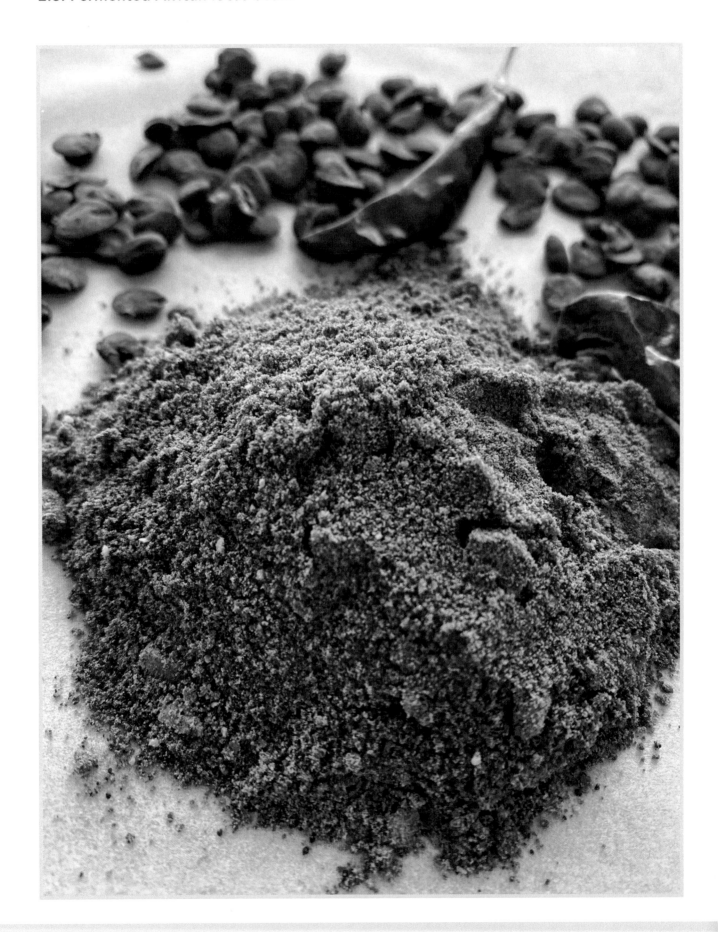

Let me introduce you to this particular bean. The locus bean isn't your ordinary bean; it comes from a towering tree up to 20 meters tall. Those trees produce large pods filled with a delightful yellow or orange pulp that's sweet and slightly dry. People enjoy it on its own or use it to make a refreshing juice too.

But the real treasure lies within the seeds enclosed in the pulp. Enter the African Locus bean, a staple in the diets of many across Central and West Africa. Imagine small, sticky, blackish balls with a fragrance that resembles the strongest cheese. The taste? Pungent and robust, giving African dishes a unique umami flavor that's unique.

This extraordinary condiment goes by different names, such as *DawaDawa*, *Soumbala*, *Nététou*, *Ugba*, or *Iru*, depending on which part of Africa you are in. This superfood has incredible taste and health benefits. So, the next time you savor the rich, umami goodness in an African dish, remember—it might just be the magic touch of the African Locus bean!

Health benefits

Packed with around 30% protein, 20% fat, 12% sugar, 15% starch, and 12% fiber, plus calcium and iron, locust bean is like a nutritional jackpot! The fermentation process adds probiotics for a gut boost. It's also a secret weapon for tackling issues like constipation, type 2 diabetes, heart disease, and colon cancer, all thanks to its fiber.

Ingredients

Dried or roasted African Locus bean
Dried chilies
Salt

Process

Just grind up all the ingredients and store that flavorful powder in a tightly sealed container. Sprinkle it into your okra, stew, greens, rice, soup, sauce, and more! Honestly, this condiment shines the most when cooked with palm oil.

You can also savor the goodness of African locust beans in their whole form—you dont have to always grind them!

3. More recipes with tropical ingredients

3.1. Palusami with palm oil or coconut oil

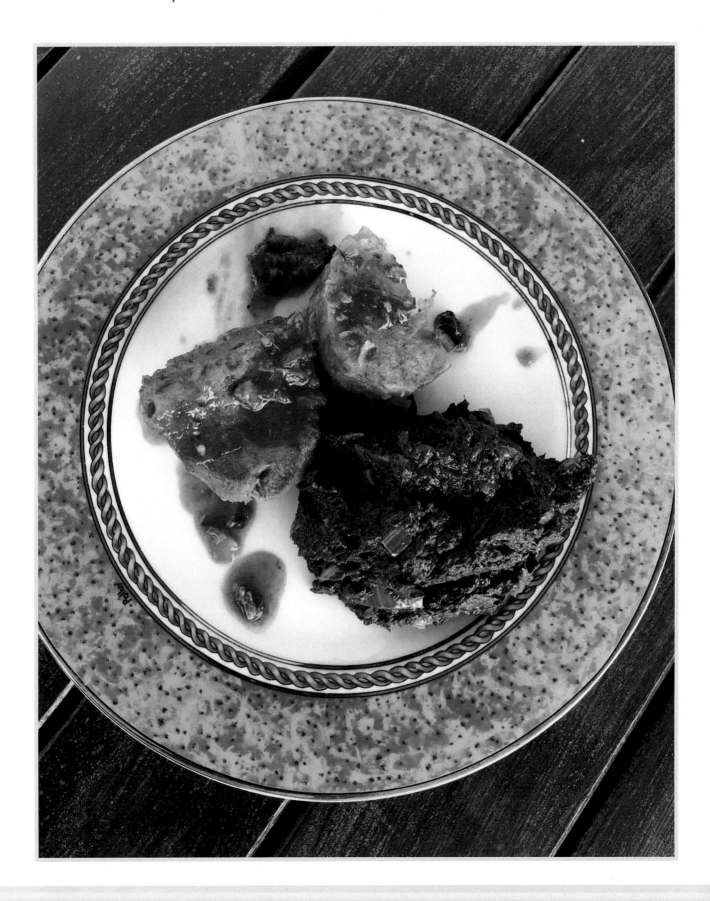

Palusami has my heart when it comes to Fijian cuisine—it's like my first culinary crush in Fiji. Made with taro leaves, coconut milk, a bit of salt, and onions, it's a simple yet perfect blend of flavors. Fijians usually enjoy it with boiled taro or cassava, and I'm all for that, but sometimes I mix it up with palm oil and a little dry crayfish for extra flavor. If I'm in the mood for something creamier, I'll add more coconut milk to make it soupier. It's also incredible with cocoyam porridge and red palm oil (see image), or really any cooked tuber.

Health benefits:

The health benefits are off the charts! Taro leaves, coconut oil or red palm oil if you prefer, and crayfish are packed with antioxidants, ready to tackle diseases head-on. They're like soldiers on your plate, standing guard against cancer and giving your heart extra love and support.

Ingredients

A bunch of Taro leaves;
1 onion
 coconut oil or palm oil;
2 tablespoons crayfish (optional);
⅓ cup of coconut milk;
salt and white pepper

Process

Start by washing the leaves thoroughly. Bring a pot of water to a boil and add the taro leaves. Let them cook uncovered for about 20 minutes. Once they're tender, strain the leaves and mash them into a paste using a fork or blender. In a separate pan, sauté onions in oil, then stir in the coconut milk and the mashed leaves. Let the mixture simmer for 5 minutes, seasoning with salt and pepper to taste. Serve this delicious dish alongside steak or roasted chicken, paired with boiled cassava, taro, or your favorite tubers.

3.2. Butter chicken

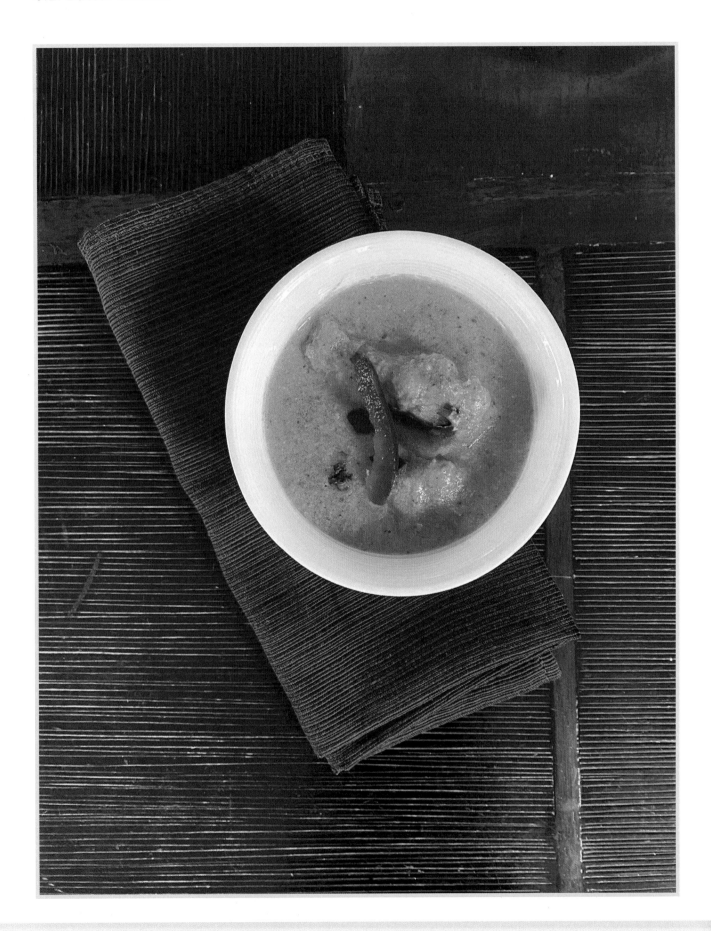

Thanks to the vibrant Indian community in Fiji, I've perfected making butter chicken from scratch. The flavor is incredible, with an explosion of spices I never knew existed. Surprisingly creamy, it's reminiscent of the African peanut sauce, *Mafé*. It pairs seamlessly with rice or hearty tubers for an ideal meal.

Health benefits

This dish follows Indian traditions, utilizing spices for flavor but also for their therapeutic benefits. Butter chicken is an undercover wellness agent, infusing a hint of spice into your life.

Ingredients

1/2 kg chicken (with or without bones)
1 tablespoon ginger and garlic paste
1 teaspoon turmeric
Half a lemon, salt

2 ½ tablespoons butter or coconut oil
1 teaspoon garam masala
1 teaspoon coriander powder
1 to 2 hot peppers
1 onion

1 cup bone stock or water
1/4 cup cashew nuts
4 medium chopped tomatoes
¼ cup Coconut cream or whipping cream

Process

Step 1:

Marinate chicken with garlic, ginger paste, turmeric, lemon, salt, coconut oil, garam masala, coriander powder, and red chili. Let it marinate for about an hour.

Step 2:

In another pot, add butter or coconut oil. Sauté onions, peeled/chopped tomatoes, add water or bone stock, cashew nuts, and boil for about 10 minutes. Allow it to cool, then blend it into a smooth paste.

Step 3:

Add butter or coconut oil to another pot. Stir in the marinated chicken over low heat until cooked.

Step 4:

Add the paste from Step 2 into the cooked chicken of step 3. Cook for additional minutes, adjusting the sauce consistency by adding bone stock or water if needed. Towards the end, add whipping cream or coconut cream. Allow it to simmer briefly before turning off the heat.

Enjoy with rice, boiled plantain, or any tuber.

3.3. Pumpkin pancakes

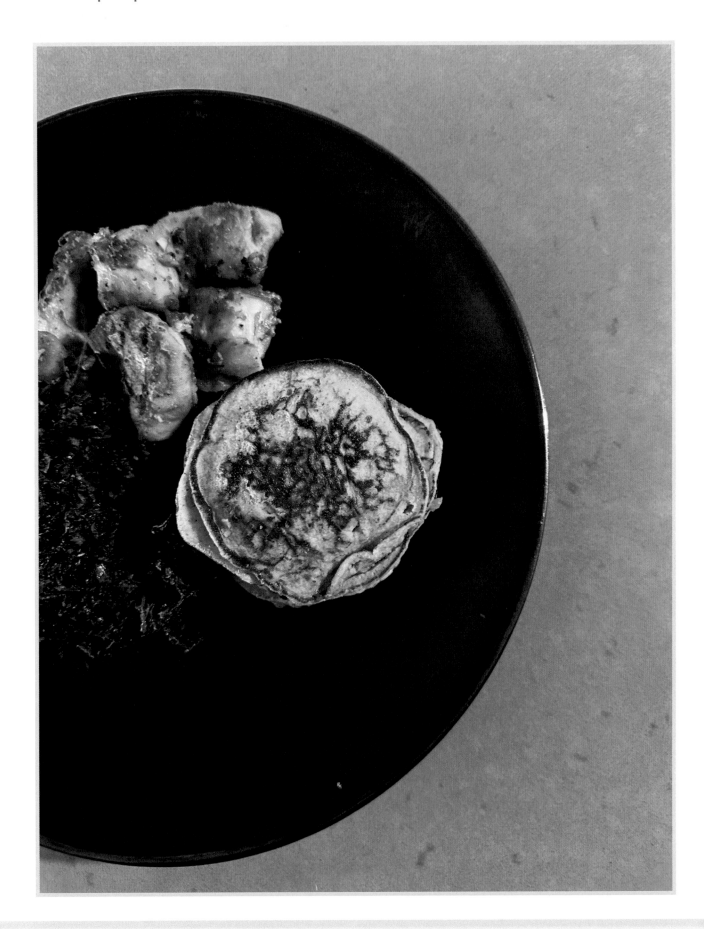

Craving a savory and nutritious pancake? Look no further—this recipe has you covered! It features almond meal, pumpkin, coconut oil, and a mix of herbs and aromatic spices. And the best part? It's gluten-free and lactose-free.

Health benefits

This savory delight is packed with aromatic herbs and spices that deliver an anti-inflammatory and antioxidant boost. Plus, you get a double dose of goodness with the healthy fats from coconut oil and almond meal.

Ingredients

4 eggs lightly beaten;
2 tablespoons almond meal
¼ cup pumpkin puree
1 teaspoon cinnamon
¼ teaspoon baking soda
¼ teaspoon ground ginger

¼ teaspoon ground nutmeg
⅛ teaspoon ground cloves
¼ teaspoon salt
¼ teaspoon white pepper
¼ teaspoon hot pepper (optional)
1½ tablespoon coconut oil

Process

Cut the pumpkin into 2 then remove all the seeds. Bake in the oven until soft. Then peel the pumpkin and mix the flesh in a blender until smooth.

Mix eggs in a bowl. Add almond meal, pumpkin, and vanilla. Stir to combine well. Mix in baking soda, spices, and salt.

Heat a pan, add the coconut oil and allow to melt. Stir the oil into the pancake mixture, leaving just a little to use for cooking pancakes.

Cook pancake until bubbles form on top, then flip and cook another minute.

You can enjoy it with grilled meat or fish or as a meal on its own. I enjoy mine with some *Nzap lah* and grilled chicken.

Source: inspired by IFM 2015, Mito's food plan

3.4. Solyanka soup

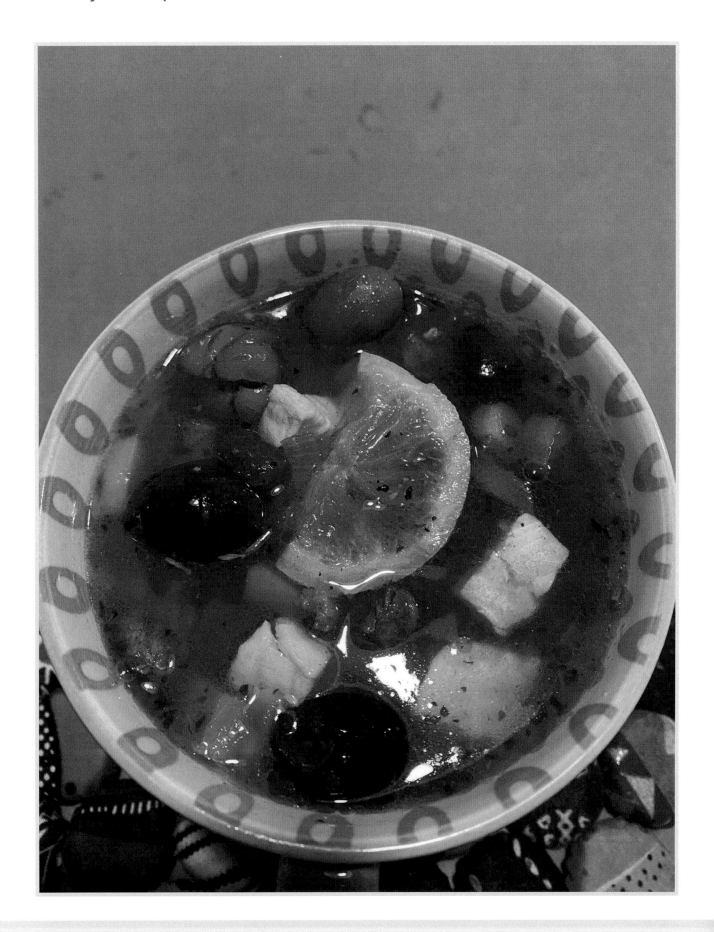

A good friend invited me for lunch and made this amazing Russian soup called Solyanka, giving me my first taste of Russian cuisine. I loved it so much that I had to return for another visit just to learn how to make it myself!

Solyanka isn't your ordinary soup. Its tangy flavor comes from salted cucumbers, pickled capers, and a dash of lemon, giving it a comforting warmth with a hint of spiciness—like a cozy hug on chilly days. Besides its unique taste, it's also said to be a great hangover cure. The best part? You can make it with fish, meat, or mushrooms, depending on your preference.

I decided to tweak the Solyanka fish recipe to fit the ingredients available in tropical countries. Forget salmon; I'm using parrot fish or snapper, whatever the local waters offer. Instead of vegetable oil, I'm going with groundnut, coconut, or avocado oil. And for an extra burst of flavor, I'm adding some locally smoked chicken or turkey.

Health benefits

This soup is packed with antioxidants from spices, fruits, and veggies, loaded with protein from the fish, and gets a healthy boost of fat from the tropical oil of your choice. Solyanka is a celebration of taste and health in a bowl!

Ingredients

1 medium onion diced
1 large carrot peeled and diced
2 potatoes peeled and cubed
150 g gherkins (salt brine cucumbers, about 6 mini ones) diced
250 g Parrot, Snapper, Tilapia, or other locally available fish
100 g smoked turkey or chicken
2 Tbsp coconut oil or avocado oil.
1 bay leaf
½ tsp black peppercorns
1 Tbsp tomato purée

1 tsp smoked paprika
1.5 liters of fish/meat stock
8 black olives quartered
8 pitted green olives quartered
1 Tbsp capers
2 Tbsp fresh lemon juice
freshly ground black pepper
1 tablespoon sliced hot pepper
2 sprigs dill finely chopped
Flat leaf parsley
4 slices of lemon

Process

In a pan over medium heat, sauté onions and carrots with a pinch of salt for approximately 4 minutes. Add tomato paste, smoked paprika, and diced gherkins (pickled cucumbers). Fry the mixture for 2 to 3 minutes.

Pour in 1.5 liters of hot homemade fish/meat stock or ready-made stock. Bring it to a boil. Add olives, capers, smoked turkey or chicken cut into bite-size chunks, and red hot peppers and cook for about 10 minutes.

Cut fresh fish (parrot/snapper) into bite-sized chunks. Add them to the soup, followed by herbs, lemon juice, and slices.

Reduce the heat to a minimum and gently poach the fish for 5 minutes. Adjust seasoning to taste. Serve the soup very hot, garnished with an extra sprinkle of fresh herbs.

Optionally, enjoy the soup with a generous chunk of fresh crunchy bread on the side. For added richness, you can incorporate coconut cream to thicken the soup and enhance the flavor.

Christine:

What started as a quest to shed some pounds turned into a transformative lifestyle through fasting and the SET-FREE method. Fast forward to today, and I'm not just witnessing weight loss; I'm living a life with increased energy levels that last all day, improved quality of sleep, and an overwhelming sense of overall well-being. Fasting became the key to unlocking a healthier and more energized version of myself!

Kola:

Navigating university life can be demanding, but introducing three days of fasting into my routine has been a game-changer. The impact on my focus and efficiency has been nothing short of remarkable. Now, I study fewer hours during fasting but get better results. Fasting has become my secret weapon for academic success, completely transforming how I approach learning!

Annex

Table 4: Carbs & Health Snapshot

	Food types	Characteristics	Impact on health
	Tropical carbs health snapshot		
Starches	Tubers like cassava, yams, cocoyams, taro or dalo, and sweet potatoes or Kumara or Boniato. Grains include millet, sorghum, teff, corn, fonio, etc.	Our body needs to break starches down into glucose to use them for energy.	<u>Source of energy</u>: Starches Provide glucose which is our body's preferred source of energy
Fibers	Soluble fiber is in beans, chickpeas, lentils or dhal, African pear, berries, avocado, cassava, etc. Insoluble fiber is in nuts, flaxseeds, peas, whole grains, wheat germ, and leafy vegetables. Unlike sugars and starches, the body doesn't digest fiber the same way. Tubers like cassava and yam are rich in both soluble and insoluble fibers.	• Soluble fibers swell in water, filling the stomach and boosting satisfaction. • Soluble fibers fuel beneficial bacteria, aiding health and growth through fermentation. • Insoluble fibers support regular and healthy stool.	• <u>Prevent obesity</u>: Filling, reducing likelihood of overeating. • <u>Prevent heart diseases</u>: Lowers risk of high cholesterol, hypertension, etc. • <u>Prevent diabetes</u>: do not spike blood sugar and insulin levels. • <u>Heal the gut</u>: Source of prebiotics, and helps reduce harmful gut bacteria.

Sugars	Fruits, milk,	These foods contain natural sugars such as glucose, lactose, and fructose. But they come with built-in sugar damage control: fibers, vitamins, and minerals in fruits; protein and fat in milk.	• <u>Source of energy</u> : Glucose feeds all cells of the body; lactose gets converted into glucose for energy use. Fructose cannot be utilized by the body cells.

Added sugar- Processed carbs health snapshot			
Processed carbs	Sugar is in most processed foods like cakes, sodas, baked goods, puff puff, mandazi, chapati, Bila, Ivy, desserts, caramelized nuts, fruits dipped in syrup, etc.	• Spikes blood sugar • High in salt, • Can be addictive due to sugars.	• <u>Feed diseases:</u> Linked to chronic diseases like cancer, heart diseases, Type 2 diabetes. • <u>Promote weight gain:</u> encourage overeating, cravings , and food addiction. • <u>Promote belly fat:</u> contribute to your "beer belly" and " menopause belly"
Added sugars	White, brown or raw sugars, Marple and agave syrups, other syrup, sweeteners, molasse, dextrose, fructose, fruit nectars, glucose, high-fructose corn syrup, lactose, malt syrup, maltose, molasses, sucrose, corn sweeteners, hydrolyzed starch, inverted sugar, palm syrup, and rice syrup, etc.		

References

Chapter I: Nutrition and lifestyle falls apart in Africa, the Caribbean and the Pacific

Asian Development Bank. (2017). *The imminent obesity crisis in Asia and the Pacific: first cost estimates* (No. 743). Retrieved from https://www.adb.org/sites/default/files/publication/320411/adbi-wp743.pdf

Bobiş, O., Dezmirean, D. S., & Moise, A. R. (2018). Honey and Diabetes: The Importance of Natural Simple Sugars in Diet for Preventing and Treating Different Types of Diabetes. *Oxidative Medicine and Cellular Longevity*, 2018, 4757893. https://doi.org/10.1155/2018/4757893.

Busnatu, S. S., et al. (2022). The Role of Fructose as a Cardiovascular Risk Factor: An Update. *Metabolites*, 12(1), 67. https://doi.org/10.3390/metabo12010067.

Fuhrman, J. (2018). The Hidden Dangers of Fast and Processed Food. *American Journal of Lifestyle Medicine*, 12(5), 375-381. https://doi.org/10.1177/1559827618766483.

Fung, J., & Moore, J. (2016). *The Complete Guide to Fasting: Heal Your Body Through Intermittent, Alternate-Day, and Extended Fasting.* Victoria: Belt Publishing Inc.

Lembke, A. (2021). *Dopamine Nation: Finding Balance in the Age of Indulgence.* Penguin Publishing Group.

Ludwig, D. S., Hu, F. B., Tappy, L., & Brand-Miller, J. (2018). Dietary carbohydrates: role of quality and quantity in chronic disease. *BMJ*, 361, k2340. https://doi.org/10.1136/bmj.k2340

McRae, M. P. (2017). Dietary Fiber Is Beneficial for the Prevention of Cardiovascular Disease: An Umbrella Review of Meta-analyses. *Journal of Chiropractic Medicine*, 16(4), 289-299. https://doi.org/10.1016/j.jcm.2017.05.005.

Nabeshima, E. H., Moro, T. M. A., Campelo, P. H., Sant'Ana, A. S., & Clerici, M. T. P. S. (2020). Tubers and roots as a source of prebiotic fibers. *Advances in Food and Nutrition Research*, 94, 267-293. https://doi.org/10.1016/bs.afnr.2020.06.005.

Pereira, R. M., et al. (2017). Fructose Consumption in the Development of Obesity and the Effects of Different Protocols of Physical Exercise on the Hepatic Metabolism. *Nutrients*, 9(4), 405. https://doi.org/10.3390/nu9040405.

Wilcox, G. (2005). Insulin and insulin resistance. *Clinical Biochemistry Reviews*, 26(2), 19-39. PMID: 16278749; PMCID: PMC1204764.

World Health Organization. (2022). Obesity rising in Africa: WHO analysis finds. Retrieved from https://www.afro.who.int/news/obesity-rising-africa-who-analysis-finds

Wu, Y., Chen, K., Taylor, A., Whaley-Connell, A., Craig, S. S., Jamal, A., Ibdah, J., & James, R. S. (2008). Insulin resistance and cardiometabolic syndrome: Adipose tissue and skeletal muscle factors. Skeletal muscle insulin resistance: Role of inflammatory cytokines and reactive oxygen species. *American Journal of Physiology. Regulatory, Integrative and Comparative Physiology*, 294(3), R673-R680. https://doi.org/10.1152/ajpregu.00561.2007

Yaribeygi, H., Maleki, M., Butler, A. E., Jamialahmadi, T., & Sahebkar, A. (2022). Molecular mechanisms linking stress and insulin resistance. *EXCLI Journal*, 21, 317-334. https://doi.org/10.17179/excli2021-4382.

Chapter III : the SET FREE method.

Traditional food

Adazabra, A. N., Ntiforo, A., & Bamford, S. A. (2014). Analysis of essential elements in Pito—a cereal food drink and its brands by the single-comparator method of neutron activation analysis. Food Science & Nutrition, 2(3), 230-235. https://doi.org/10.1002/fsn3.95. Epub 2014 Mar 5. PMID: 24936292; PMCID: PMC4048608.

Aalbersberg, W. G. L., Lovelace, C. E. A., Madhoji, K., & Parkinson, S. V. (2010). Davuke, the traditional Fijian method of pit preservation of staple carbohydrate foods. In *Pages 173-180*. https://doi.org/10.1080/03670244.1988.9991030.

Barampama, Z., & Simard, R. E. (1995). Effects of soaking, cooking, and fermentation on composition, in-vitro starch digestibility, and nutritive value of common beans. Plant Foods for Human Nutrition, 48(4), 349-365. https://doi.org/10.1007/BF01088494.

Barak, S., & Mudgil, D. (2014). Locust bean gum: Processing, properties, and food applications—a review. International Journal of Biological Macromolecules, 66, 74-80. https://doi.org/10.1016/j.ijbiomac.2014.02.017. Epub 2014 Feb 16. PMID: 24548746.

Borojevic, K., & Borojevic, K. (2005). The transfer and history of "Reduced Height Genes" (Rht) in wheat from Japan to Europe. Journal of Heredity, 96(4), 455–459. https://doi.org/10.1093/jhered/esi060

Centre for Food Safety. (2008, February). Food Safety Focus (19th Issue) – Incident in Focus: Cyanide Poisoning and Cassava. Reported by Ms. Joey Kwok, Scientific Officer, Risk Communication Section. https://www.cfs.gov.hk/english/multimedia/multimedia_pub/multimedia_pub_fsf_19_01.html#:~:text=Sweet%20cassava%20roots%20contain%20less,by%20peeling%20and%20thorough%20cooking.

Chandrasekara, A., & Josheph Kumar, T. (2016). Roots and tuber crops as functional foods: A review on phytochemical constituents and their potential health benefits. International Journal of Food Science, 2016, 3631647. https://doi.org/10.1155/2016/3631647.

Chu, J. (2015, September). Risk Assessment Section. Center for Food Safety: The Government of the Hong Kong Special Administrative Region. Food Safety Focus (110th Issue) – Incident in Focus. Cyanides and Food Safety.

Diaz, M., Sayavedra, L., Atter, A., Mayer, M. J., Saha, S., Amoa-Awua, W., & Narbad, A. (2020). Lactobacillus garii sp. nov., isolated from a fermented cassava product. International Journal of Systematic and Evolutionary Microbiology, 70(5), 3012-3017. https://doi.org/10.1099/ijsem.0.004121

Erukainure, O. L., Oyebode, O. A., Chukwuma, C. I., Matsabisa, M. G., Koorbanally, N. A., & Islam, M. S. (2019). Raffia palm (Raphia hookeri) wine inhibits glucose diffusion; improves antioxidative activities; and modulates dysregulated pathways and metabolites in oxidative pancreatic injury. Journal of Food Biochemistry, 43(3), e12749. https://doi.org/10.1111/jfbc.12749. Epub 2018 Dec 17. PMID: 31353563.

FFTC. (n.d.). Processing cassava into flour for human. FFTC Practical Technology. https://www.fftc.org.tw/htmlarea_file/library/20110716232822/pt2003017.pdf

Food and Agriculture Organization (FAO). (2005). Proceedings of the Validation Forum on the Global Cassava Development Strategy, Volume 2: A review of cassava in Africa with country case studies on Nigeria, Ghana, the United Republic of Tanzania, Uganda and Benin. International Fund for Agricultural Development, Food and Agriculture Organization of the United Nations, Rome. Retrieved from https://www.fao.org/3/a0154e/a0154e.pdf

Fung, J. (2016). The Obesity Code: Unlocking the Secret of Weight Loss. Greystones Books.

Fung, J. (2018). The Diabetes Code: Prevent and Reverse Type 2 Diabetes Naturally. Greystones Books.

Fung, J., & Moore, J. (2016). The Complete Guide to Fasting: Heal Your Body Through Intermittent, Alternate-Day, and Extended Fasting. Victoria: Belt Publishing Inc.

González, R., Ballester, I., López-Posadas, R., Suárez, M. D., Zarzuelo, A., Martínez-Augustin, O., & Sánchez de Medina, F. (2011). Effects of flavonoids and other polyphenols on inflammation. Critical Reviews in Food Science and Nutrition, 51(4), 331-362. https://doi.org/10.1080/10408390903584094. PMID: 21432698.

Gopalakrishnan, L., Doriya, K., & Kumar, D. S. (2016). Moringa oleifera: A review on nutritive importance and its medicinal application. Food Science and Human Wellness, 5(2), 49-56. https://doi.org/10.1016/j.fshw.2016.04.001

Hano, C., & Tungmunnithum, D. (2020). Plant Polyphenols, More than Just Simple Natural Antioxidants: Oxidative Stress, Aging and Age-Related Diseases. Medicines (Basel), 7(5), 26. https://doi.org/10.3390/medicines7050026.

Hano, C., & Tungmunnithum, D. (2020). Plant Polyphenols, More than Just Simple Natural Antioxidants: Oxidative Stress, Aging and Age-Related Diseases. Medicines (Basel), 7(5), 26. https://doi.org/10.3390/medicines7050026.

Jiang, C., Li, G., Huang, P., Liu, Z., & Zhao, B. (2017). The gut microbiota and Alzheimer's disease. Journal of Alzheimer's Disease, 58(1), 1-15. https://doi.org/10.3233/JAD-161141. PMID: 28372330.

Kim, T. K., Yong, H. I., Kim, Y. B., Kim, H. W., & Choi, Y. S. (2019). Edible insects as a protein source: A review of public perception, processing technology, and research trends. Food Science of Animal Resources, 39(4), 521-540. https://doi.org/10.5851/kosfa.2019.e53. Epub 2019 Aug 31. PMID: 31508584; PMCID: PMC6728817.

Khatun, H., Rahman, A., Biswas, M., & Islam, A. U. (2011). Water-soluble fraction of Abelmoschus esculentus (Okra) L interacts with glucose and metformin hydrochloride and alters their absorption kinetics after coadministration in rats. https://doi.org/10.5402/2011/260537.

Kuete, V. (2017). Medicinal spices and vegetables from Africa. Chapter 13 - Other health benefits of African medicinal spices and vegetables. In Therapeutic Potential Against

Li, W. (2019). Eat to Beat Disease: The Body's Five Defense Systems and the Food That Can Save Your Life. Vermilion, Hachette Book Group.

Metabolic, Inflammatory, Infectious and Systemic Diseases (pp. 329-349). Academic Press. Editor(s): Victor Kuete. https://doi.org/10.1016/B978-0-12-809286-6.00013-3

Nangula, P. U., et al. (2010). Nutritional value of leafy vegetables of sub-Saharan Africa and their potential contribution to human health: A review. *Journal of Food Composition and Analysis, 23*(6), 499-509. https://doi.org/10.1016/j.jfca.2010.05.002.

National Research Council (US) Committee on Diet and Health. (1989). *Diet and Health: Implications for Reducing Chronic Disease Risk* (11, Fat-Soluble Vitamins). Washington, DC: National Academies Press. Available from: https://www.ncbi.nlm.nih.gov/books/NBK218749/

Obafemi, Y. D., Oranusi, S. U., Ajanaku, K. O., Akinduti, P. A., Leech, J., & Cotter, P. D. (2022). African fermented foods: Overview, emerging benefits, and novel approaches to microbiome profiling. *NPJ Science of Food, 6*(1), 15. https://doi.org/10.1038/s41538-022-00130-w

Obrenovich, M. E. M. (2018). Leaky Gut, Leaky Brain? *Microorganisms, 6*(4), 107. https://doi.org/10.3390/microorganisms6040107. PMID: 30340384; PMCID: PMC6313445.

Ogbuonye, E. O. (2018). Chemical and microbial evaluation of 'Ogiri' (a locally fermented food condiment) produced from Kersting groundnut seeds. *Science Arena Publication, Specialty Journal of Biological Sciences, Department of Food Technology, Federal Polytechnic, Oko, Anambra State, Nigeria, 4*(2), 7-13. Available online at www.sciarena.com.

Olajugbagbe, T. E., Elugbadebo, O. E., & Omafuvbe, B. O. (2020). Probiotic potentials of Pediococcus acidilactici isolated from wara: A Nigerian unripened soft cheese. *Heliyon, 6*(9), e04889. https://doi.org/10.1016/j.heliyon.2020.e04889.

Padmaja, G. (1995). Cyanide detoxification in cassava for food and feed uses. *Critical Reviews in Food Science and Nutrition, 35*(4), 299-339. https://doi.org/10.1080/10408399509527703. PMID: 7576161.

Page Islam, Z., Islam, S. M. R., Hossen, F., Mahtab-Ul-Islam, K., Hasan, M. R., & Karim, R. (2021). *Moringa oleifera is a prominent source of nutrients with potential health benefits. International Journal of Food Science,* 2021, 6627265. https://doi.org/10.1155/2021/6627265

Pandey, K. B., & Rizvi, S. I. (2009). Plant polyphenols as dietary antioxidants in human health and disease. *Oxidative Medicine and Cellular Longevity, 2*(5), 270-278. https://doi.org/10.4161/oxim.2.5.9498. PMID: 20716914; PMCID: PMC2835915.

Petersen, C., & Round, J. L. (2014). Defining dysbiosis and its influence on host immunity and disease. *Cell Microbiology, 16*(7), 1024-1033. https://doi.org/10.1111/cmi.12308. Epub 2014 Jun 2. PMID: 24798552; PMCID: PMC4143175.

Poulain, M., Herm, A., & Pes, G. (2013). The Blue Zones: Areas of exceptional longevity around the world. *Vienna Yearbook of Population Research, 11*, 87–108. doi:10.1553/populationyearbook2013s87

Rahimzadeh, M. R., Rahimzadeh, M. R., Kazemi, S., Amiri, R. J., Pirzadeh, M., & Moghadamnia, A. A. (2022). Aluminum poisoning with emphasis on its mechanism and treatment of intoxication. *Emergency Medicine International, 2022*, 1480553. https://doi.org/10.1155/2022/1480553.

Rietman, A., Schwarz, J., Tomé, D., Kok, F. J., & Mensink, M. (2014). High dietary protein intake, reducing or eliciting insulin resistance? *European Journal of Clinical Nutrition, 68*(9), 973-979. https://doi.org/10.1038/ejcn.2014.123. Epub 2014 Jul 2. PMID: 24986822.

Sarker, U., Hossain, M. M., & Oba, S. (2020). Nutritional and antioxidant components and antioxidant capacity in green morph Amaranthus leafy vegetable. *Scientific Reports, 10*(1), 1336. https://doi.org/10.1038/s41598-020-57687-3. PMID: 31992722; PMCID: PMC6987210.

Shanahan, C., & Shanahan, L. (2009). *Deep Nutrition: Why Your Genes Need Traditional Food.* Big Box Books.

Suter, P. M., Schutz, Y., & Jequier, E. (1992). The effect of ethanol on fat storage in healthy subjects. *New England Journal of Medicine, 326*(15), 983-987. https://doi.org/10.1056/NEJM199204093261503. PMID: 1545851.

Uchechukwu, I., et al. (2018). Nutritional composition and antinutritional properties of maize ogi cofermented with pigeon pea. *Food Science and Nutrition Articles.* https://doi.org/10.1002/fsn3.571.

University of Hawai'i at Manoa Library. (n.d.). *Traditional Pacific Island Crops: Cassava.* https://guides.library.manoa.hawaii.edu/paccrops/cassava#:~:text=Cassava%20was%20introduced%20to%20the,produced%20on%20a%20large%20scale

Wang, C., Murgia, M. A., Baptista, J., et al. (2022). Sardinian dietary analysis for longevity: A review of the literature. *Journal of Ethnic Foods, 9*, 33. https://doi.org/10.1186/s42779-022-00152-5

Wu, X., Qian, L., Liu, K., Wu, J., & Shan, Z. (2021). Gastrointestinal microbiome and gluten in celiac disease. *Annals of Medicine, 53*(1), 1797-1805. https://doi.org/10.1080/07853890.2021.1990392. PMID: 34647492; PMCID:

Xu, T., Huang, W., Liang, J., Zhong, Y., Chen, Q., Jie, F., & Lu, B. (2021). Tuber flours improve intestinal health and modulate gut microbiota composition. *Food Chemistry X, 12*, 100145. https://doi.org/10.1016/j.fochx.2021.100145. PMID: 34765968; PMCID: PMC8571703.

Yan, L. (2013). Dark green leafy vegetables. *Agriculture Research Service, United States Department of Agriculture.* https://www.ars.usda.gov/plains-area/gfnd/gfhnrc/docs/news-2013/dark-green-leafy-vegetables#:~:text=They%20also%20contain%20high%20levels,helps%20prevent%20certain%20birth%20defects.

Yang, X., Darko, K. O., Huang, Y., He, C., Yang, H., He, S., Li, J., Li, J., Hocher, B., & Yin, Y. (2017). Resistant starch regulates gut microbiota: Structure, biochemistry and cell signalling. *Cell Physiology and Biochemistry, 42*(1), 306-318. https://doi.org/10.1159/000477386. Epub 2017 May 25. PMID: 28535508.

Yen, A. L. (2015). Insects as food and feed in the Asia Pacific region: Current perspectives and future directions. *Journal of Insects as Food and Feed, 1*(1), 33-55. Department of Economic Development, Jobs, Transport and Resources, Biosciences Research Division, AgriBio, 5 Ring Road, Bundoora, Victoria 3083, Australia; La Trobe University, School of Applied Systems Biology, AgriBio, 5 Ring Road, Bundoora, Victoria 3083, Wageningen Academic Publishers.

Fat and Tropical Cooking oil : Red Palm oil , coconut oil and groundnut oi

Arya, S. S., Salve, A. R., & Chauhan, S. (2016). Peanuts as functional food: a review. Journal of Food Science and Technology, 53(1), 31-41. doi: 10.1007/s13197-015-2007-9. PMID: 26787930; PMCID: PMC4711439.

Bishop, T., & Figueredo, V. M. (2001). Hypertensive therapy: Attacking the renin-angiotensin system. Western Journal of Medicine, 175(2), 119-124. doi: 10.1136/ewjm.175.2.119. PMID: 11483557; PMCID: PMC1071503.

Boateng, L., Ansong, R., Owusu, W. B., & Steiner-Asiedu, M. (2016). Coconut oil and palm oil's role in nutrition, health, and national development: A review. Ghana Medical Journal, 50(3), 189-196. PMID: 27752194; PMCID: PMC5044790.

Canfield, L. M., Kaminsky, R. G., Taren, D. L., Shaw, E., & Sander, J. K. (2001). Red palm oil in the maternal diet increases provitamin A carotenoids in breastmilk and serum of the mother-infant dyad. European Journal of Nutrition, 40(1), 30-38. https://doi.org/10.1007/pl00007383. PMID: 11315503.

Edem, D. O. (2002). Palm oil: Biochemical, physiological, nutritional, hematological, and toxicological aspects: A review. Plant Foods for Human Nutrition, 57(3-4), 319-341. https://doi.org/10.1023/a:1021828132707. PMID: 12602939.

Fattore, E., Bosetti, C., Brighenti, F., Agostoni, C., & Fattore, G. (2014). Palm oil and blood lipid-related markers of cardiovascular disease: A systematic review and meta-analysis of dietary intervention trials. American Journal of Clinical Nutrition, 99(6), 1331-1350. https://doi.org/10.3945/ajcn.113.081190. Epub 2014 Apr 9. PMID: 24717342.

Feldman, E. B. (1999). Assorted monounsaturated fatty acids promote healthy hearts. The American Journal of Clinical Nutrition, 70(6), 953-954. https://doi.org/10.1093/ajcn/70.6.953.

German, J. B., & Dillard, C. J. (2010). Saturated fats: A perspective from lactation and milk composition. *Lipids, 45*(10), 915-923. https://doi.org/10.1007/s11745-010-3445-9. Epub 2010 Jul 23.

Hewlings, S. (2020). Coconuts and Health: Different Chain Lengths of Saturated Fats Require Different Consideration. Journal of Cardiovascular Development and Disease, 7(4), 59. doi: 10.3390/jcdd7040059. PMID: 33348586; PMCID: PMC7766932.

James, J., & James, H. O. (2018). Omega-6 vegetable oils as a driver of coronary heart disease: The oxidized linoleic acid hypothesis. BMJ Open Heart, 5(2). http://dx.doi.org/10.1136/openhrt-2018-000898.

Lucci, P., et al. (2016). Palm oil and cardiovascular disease: A randomized trial of the effects of hybrid palm oil supplementation on human plasma lipid patterns. Food Function, 7(1), 347-354. https://doi.org/10.1039/c5fo01083g. PMID: 26488229.

Loganathan, R., Subramaniam, K. M., Radhakrishnan, A. K., Choo, Y.-M., Teng, K.-T., & Tiu, K.-M. (2017). Health-promoting effects of red palm oil: Evidence from animal and human studies. Nutrition Reviews, 75(2), 98–113. https://doi.org/10.1093/nutrit/nuw054.

Malhotra, A., Redberg, R. F., & Meier, P. (2017). Saturated fat does not clog the arteries: Coronary heart disease is a chronic inflammatory condition, the risk of which can be effectively reduced from healthy lifestyle interventions. British Journal of Sports Medicine, 51(15), 1111-1112. doi: 10.1136/bjsports-2016-097285.

Marcus, J. B. (2013). Lipids Basics: Fats and Oils in Foods and Health; Tropical oils. Culinary Nutrition. Retrieved from https://www.sciencedirect.com/topics/neuroscience/coconut-oil.

Mojtaba, Y., & Hedayat, H. (n.d.). Evaluation of Hexane Content in Edible Vegetable Oils Consumed in Iran. Food Safety Research Center (Salt), School of Nutrition and Food Sciences, Semnan University of Medical Sciences, Semnan, Iran. Department of Food Science and Technology, Faculty of Nutrition Sciences, Food Science and Technology/National Nutrition and Food Technology Research Institute, Shahid Beheshti University of Medical Sciences, Tehran, Iran. DOI 10.14302/issn.2641-7669.ject-17-1790.

McGee, D., Reed, D., Stemmerman, G., Rhoads, G., Yano, K., & Feinleib, M. (1985). The relationship of dietary fat and cholesterol to mortality in 10 years: The Honolulu Heart Program. International Journal of Epidemiology, 14(1), 97-105. doi: 10.1093/ije/14.1.97.

Mumme, K., & Stonehouse, W. (2015). Effects of medium-chain triglycerides on weight loss and body composition: a meta-analysis of randomized controlled trials. Journal of the Academy of Nutrition and Dietetics, 115(2), 249-263. doi: 10.1016/j.jand.2014.10.022. PMID: 25636220.

Oglesby, P. (n.d.). Chicago Western Electric Study: The Cohort Study (1947-1972). Heart Attack Prevention: A History of Cardiovascular Disease Epidemiology. Year Begun: 1957. Illinois, USA. http://www.epi.umn.edu/cvdepi/study-synopsis/chicago-western-electric-study/.

Oguntibeju, O. O., Esterhuyse, A. J., & Truter, E. J. (2009). Red palm oil: Nutritional, physiological, and therapeutic roles in improving human wellbeing and quality of life. *British Journal of Biomedical Science, 66*(4), 216-222. https://doi.org/10.1080/09674845.2009.11730279. PMID: 20095133.

O'Donnell, C. J., & Elosua, R. (2008). Cardiovascular Risk Factors. Insights From Framingham Heart Study. National Heart, Lung and Blood Institute's Cardiology Division, Department of Medicine, Massachusetts General Hospital, Harvard Medical School, Boston.

Rachaputi, R.C.N., & Wright, G. (2016). Peanuts, Overview. *Reference Module in Food Science.* Elsevier. https://www.sciencedirect.com/science/article/abs/pii/B978008100596500038X

Soedamah-Muthu, S. S., Masset, G., Verberne, L., Geleijnse, J. M., & Brunner, E. J. (2013). Consumption of dairy products and associations with incident diabetes, CHD and mortality in the Whitehall II study. British Journal of Nutrition, 109(4), 718-726. doi: 10.1017/S0007114512001845.

Teicholz, N. (2023). A short history of saturated fat: the making and unmaking of a scientific consensus. *Current Opinion in Endocrinology, Diabetes, and Obesity, 30*(1), 65-71. https://doi.org/10.1097/MED.0000000000000791. Epub 2022 Dec 8. PMID: 36477384; PMCID: PMC9794145.

Tham, E. H., & Leung, D. Y. M. (2018). How Different Parts of the World Provide New Insights Into Food Allergy. *Allergy Asthma Immunol Res*, 10(4), 290-299. https://doi.org/10.4168/aair.2018.10.4.290

Voon, P. T., Ng, T. K., Lee, V. K., & Nesaretnam, K. (2015). Virgin olive oil, palm olein, and coconut oil diets do not raise cell adhesion molecules and thrombogenicity indices in healthy Malaysian adults. *European Journal of Clinical Nutrition, 69*(6), 712-716. https://doi.org/10.1038/ejcn.2015.26. Epub 2015 Mar 25. PMID: 25804278.

Wattanapenpaiboon, N., & Wahlqvist, M. W. (2003). Phytonutrient deficiency: The place of palm fruit. *Asia Pacific Journal of Clinical Nutrition, 12*(3), 363-368. PMID: 14506002.

Yuan, M., Singer, M. R., Pickering, R. T., & Moore, L. L. (2022). Saturated fat from dairy sources is associated with lower cardiometabolic risk in the Framingham Offspring Study. *American Journal of Clinical Nutrition, 116*(6), 1682-1692. https://doi.org/10.1093/ajcn/nqac224. PMID: 36307959; PMCID: PMC9761752.

Dare to borrow ideas

Mikami, K., & Hosokawa, M. (2013). Biosynthetic pathway and health benefits of fucoxanthin, an algae-specific xanthophyll in brown seaweeds. *International Journal of Molecular Sciences, 14*(7), 13763-13781. https://doi.org/10.3390/ijms140713763

Peñalver, R., Lorenzo, J. M., Ros, G., Amarowicz, R., Pateiro, M., & Nieto, G. (2020). Seaweeds as a functional ingredient for a healthy diet. *Marine Drugs, 18*(6), 301. https://doi.org/10.3390/md18060301

Intermittent fasting

Albosta, M., & Bakke, J. (2021). Intermittent fasting: Is there a role in the treatment of diabetes? A review of the literature and guide for primary care physicians. Clinic Diabetes Endocrinology. https://doi.org/10.1186/s40842-020-00116-1

Anton, S. D., et al. (2018). Flipping the metabolic switch: Understanding and applying the health benefits of fasting. Obesity, A Research Journal, 26(2), 254-268. https://doi.org/10.1002/oby.22065

As-Badrani, S. M., & others. (2022). Consequences of Insulin Resistance Long Term in the Body and Its Association with the Development of Chronic Diseases. Journal of Bioscience and Medicine, 10(12). DOI: 10.4236/jbm.2022.1012009.

Bagheriya, M., Butler, A. E., Barreto, G. E., & Sahebkar, A. (2018). The effect of fasting or calorie restriction on autophagy induction: A review of the literature. Ageing Research Reviews, 47, 183-197. https://doi.org/10.1016/j.arr.2018.08.004.

Bastani, A., Rajabi, S., & Kianimarkani, F. (2017). The Effects of Fasting During Ramadan on the Concentration of Serotonin, Dopamine, Brain-Derived Neurotrophic Factor, and Nerve Growth Factor. Neurol Int, 9(2), 7043. doi: 10.4081/ni.2017.7043

Cignarella, F., Cantoni, C., Ghezzi, L., et al. (2018). Intermittent fasting confers protection in CNS autoimmunity by altering the gut microbiota. Cell Metabolism, 27(6), 1222-1235.e6. doi: 10.1016/j.cmet.2018.05.006

Drenick, E. J., Swendseid, M. E., Blahd, W. H., & Tuttle, S. G. (1964). Prolonged starvation as treatment for severe obesity. *JAMA, 187*, 100-105. https://doi.org/10.1001/jama.1964.03060150024006

Fung, J., & Moore, J. (2016). The complete guide to fasting: Heal your body through intermittent, alternate-day, and extended fasting. Victoria: Belt Publishing Inc.

Freeman, A. M., & Pennings, N. (2022). Insulin Resistance. National Library of Medicine. National Center for Biotechnology Information. NIH. Retrieved July 2023 from https://www.ncbi.nlm.nih.gov/books/NBK507839/

Goldenberg, N., Horowitz, J. F., Gorgey, A., et al. (2022). Role of pulsatile growth hormone (GH) secretion in the regulation of lipolysis in fasting humans. Clinical Diabetes Endocrinology, 8, 1. https://doi.org/10.1186/s40842-022-00137-y

Goodpaster, B. H., & Sparks, L. M. (2017). Metabolic flexibility in health and disease. *Cell Metabolism, 25*(5), 1027-1036. https://doi.org/10.1016/j.cmet.2017.04.015

Hartman, M. L., Veldhuis, J. D., Johnson, M. L., Lee, M. M., Alberti, K. G., Samojlik, E., & Thorner, M. O. (1992). Augmented growth hormone (GH) secretory burst frequency and amplitude mediate enhanced GH secretion during a two-day fast in normal men. Journal of Clinical Endocrinology & Metabolism, 74(4), 757-765. https://doi.org/10.1210/jcem.74.4.1548337

Hintz, R. L. (2004). Growth hormone: Uses and abuses. BMJ, 328(7445), 907-908. https://doi.org/10.1136/bmj.328.7445.907

Lettieri-Barbato, D., Cannata, S. M., Casagrande, V., Ciriolo, M. R., & Aquilano, K. (2018). Time-controlled fasting prevents aging-like mitochondrial changes induced by persistent dietary fat overload in skeletal muscle. PLoS One, 13(5), e0195912. https://doi.org/10.1371/journal.pone.0195912

Lettieri-Barbato, D., et al. (2020). Fasting Drives Nrf2-Related Antioxidant Response in Skeletal Muscle. International Journal of Molecular Sciences, 21(20), 7780. https://doi.org/10.3390/ijms21207780.

Lilja, S., Stoll, C., Krammer, U., et al. (2021). Five days periodic fasting elevates levels of longevity-related Christensenella and sirtuin expression in humans. International Journal of Molecular Sciences, 22(5), 2331. doi: 10.3390/ijms22052331

Malinowski, B., et al. (2019). Intermittent Fasting in Cardiovascular Disorders—An Overview. Nutrients, 11(3), 673. https://doi.org/10.3390/nu11030673.

Mager, D. E., Wan, R., Brown, M., Cheng, A., Wareski, P., Abernethy, D. R., & Mattson, M. P. (2006). Caloric restriction and intermittent fasting alter spectral measures of heart rate and blood pressure variability in rats. FASEB Journal, 20(5), 631–637. [CrossRef]

Mateos-Aparicio, P., & Rodríguez-Moreno, A. (2019). The impact of studying brain plasticity. *Frontiers in Cellular Neuroscience, 13*, 66. [PMC free article] [PubMed]

Mattson, M. P., Moehl, K., Ghena, N., Schmaedick, M., & Cheng, A. (2018). Intermittent metabolic switching, neuroplasticity and brain health. Nature Reviews Neuroscience, 19(2), 63-80. https://

doi.org/10.1038/nrn.2017.156 Erratum in: Nature Reviews Neuroscience, 21(8), 445. https://doi.org/10.1038/s41583-020-0331-3

NHS. (2022, September). Stem cells and bone marrow transplants. Retrieved from https://www.nhs.uk/conditions/stem-cell-transplant/risks/

Palmer, B. F., & Clegg, D. J. (2022). Metabolic flexibility and its impact on health outcomes. Mayo Clinic Proceedings, 97(4), 761-776. https://doi.org/10.1016/j.mayocp.2022.01.012.

Pallauf, K., & Rimbach, G. (2013). Autophagy, polyphenols and healthy ageing. Ageing Research Reviews, 12(1), 237-252. https://doi.org/10.1016/j.arr.2012.03.008.

Sutton, E. F., et al. (2018). Early Time-Restricted Feeding Improves Insulin Sensitivity, Blood Pressure, and Oxidative Stress Even without Weight Loss in Men with Prediabetes. Cell Metabolism, 27(6), 1212-1221.e3. doi: 10.1016/j.cmet.2018.04.010

Walsh, J. J., Edgett, B. A., Tschakovsky, M. E., & Gurd, B. J. (2015). Fasting and exercise differentially regulate BDNF mRNA expression in human skeletal muscle. Applied Physiology, Nutrition, and Metabolism, 40(1), 96-98. https://doi.org/10.1139/apnm-2014-0290.

Wang, H., Wang, A. X., Aylor, K., & Barrett, E. J. (2013). Nitric oxide directly promotes vascular endothelial insulin transport. Diabetes, 62(12), 4030–4042. https://doi.org/10.2337/db13-0627

Wang, S., Deng, Z., Ma, Y., et al. (2020). The role of autophagy and mitophagy in bone metabolic disorders. International Journal of Biological Sciences, 16(14), 2675-2691. https://doi.org/10.7150/ijbs.46627

Wegman, M. P., et al. (2015). Practicality of intermittent fasting in humans and its effect on oxidative stress and genes related to aging and metabolism. Rejuvenation, 18(2), 162-172. https://doi.org/10.1089/rej.2014.1624.

Wilhelmi de Toledo, F., Grundler, F., Bergouignan, A., Drinda, S., & Michalsen, A. (2019). Safety, health improvement and well-being during a 4 to 21-day fasting period in an observational study including 1422 subjects. PLoS One, 14(1), e0209353. https://doi.org/10.1371/journal.pone.0209353

Zhang, J., Xiang, H., Liu, J., Chen, Y., He, R. R., & Liu, B. (2020). Mitochondrial Sirtuin 3: New emerging biological function and therapeutic target. Theranostics, 10(18), 8315-8342. https://doi.org/10.7150/thno.45922

Zhao, Y., Jia, M., Chen, W., & Liu, Z. (2022). The neuroprotective effects of intermittent fasting on brain aging and neurodegenerative diseases via regulating mitochondrial function. Free Radical Biology & Medicine, 182, 206-218. https://doi.org/10.1016/j.freeradbiomed.2022.02.021

Routine exercise

Brattico, E., Bonetti, L., Ferretti, G., Vuust, P., & Matrone, C. (2021). Putting cells in motion: Advantages of endogenous boosting of BDNF production. *Cells, 10*(1), 183. https://doi.org/10.3390/cells10010183

MedlinePlus. (2017). Health risks of an inactive lifestyle. Also called: sedentary lifestyle, sitting disease. National Library of Medicine. https://medlineplus.gov/healthrisksofaninactivelifestyle.html#:~:text=Not%20exercising.,very%20little%20to%20no%20exercise

MedlinePlus. (2020, December). Cholesterol (also called: Hypercholesterolemia, Hyperlipidemia, Hyperlipoproteinemia). MedlinePlus. https://medlineplus.gov/cholesterol.html

Møller, A. B., Vendelbo, M. H., Christensen, B., & Clasen, B. F. (2015). Physical exercise increases autophagic signaling through ULK1 in human skeletal muscle. *Journal of Applied Physiology.* https://doi.org/10.1152/japplphysiol.01116.2014

Monda, V., Villano, I., Messina, A., Valenzano, A., Esposito, T., Moscatelli, F., Viggiano, A., Cibelli, G., Chieffi, S., Monda, M., & Messina, G. (2017). Exercise modifies the gut microbiota with positive health effects. *Oxidative Medicine and Cellular Longevity, 2017*, 3831972. https://doi.org/10.1155/2017/3831972

Pereira, R. M., et al. (2017). Fructose Consumption in the Development of Obesity and the Effects of Different Protocols of Physical Exercise on the Hepatic Metabolism. *Nutrients, 9*(4), 405. https://doi.org/10.3390/nu9040405

Be the expert in charge of your health

Bahrami, T., Rejeh, N., Heravi-Karimooi, M., Tadrisi, S. D., & Vaismoradi, M. (2019). The effect of foot reflexology on hospital anxiety and depression in female older adults: A randomized controlled trial. *International Journal of Therapeutic Massage & Bodywork, 12*(3), 16-21. https://doi.org/10.3822/ijtmb.v12i3.346

Breit, S., Kupferberg, A., Rogler, G., & Hasler, G. (2018). Vagus nerve as modulator of the brain-gut axis in psychiatric and inflammatory disorders. *Frontiers in Psychiatry, 9*, 44. https://doi.org/10.3389/fpsyt.2018.00044

Lin, J., & Epel, E. (2022). Stress and telomere shortening: Insights from cellular mechanisms. *Ageing Research Reviews, 73*, 101507. https://doi.org/10.1016/j.arr.2021.101507

NHS. (2022). Statin side effect. Retrieved from https://www.nhs.uk/conditions/statins/side-effects/#:~:text=dizziness,constipation%2C%20diarrhoea%2C%20indigestion%20or%20farting

Pavlov, V. A., & Tracey, K. J. (2012). The vagus nerve and the inflammatory reflex: Linking immunity and metabolism. *Nature Reviews Endocrinology, 8*(12), 743–754. https://doi.org/10.1038/nrendo.2012.189

Chapter IV. Health Hacks : conquer disease and own wellness

Why tea is more than just a drink

Ajuwon, O. R., Ayeleso, A. O., & Adefolaju, G. A. (2018). The potential of South African herbal tisanes, rooibos and honeybush in the management of type 2 diabetes mellitus. *Molecules, 23*(12), 3207. https://doi.org/10.3390/molecules23123207

Cancer Association of South Africa. (March 2021). Fact sheet on Honeybush tea.

Marnewick, J. L., van der Westhuizen, F. H., Joubert, E., Swanevelder, S., Swart, P., & Gelderblom, W. C. (2009). Chemoprotective properties of rooibos (Aspalathus linearis), honeybush (Cyclopia intermedia) herbal and green and black (Camellia sinensis) teas against cancer promotion induced by fumonisin B1 in rat liver. *Food and Chemical Toxicology, 47*(1), 220-229. https://doi.org/10.1016/j.fct.2008.11.004

Sissing, L., Marnewick, J., de Kock, M., Swanevelder, S., Joubert, E., & Gelderblom, W. (2011). Modulating effects of rooibos and honeybush herbal teas on the development of esophageal papillomas in rats. *Nutrition and Cancer, 63*(4), 600-610. https://doi.org/10.1080/01635581.2011.539313

Reversing T2D and Hypertension

Choi, J. W., Ford, E. S., Gao, X., & Choi, H. K. (2007). Sugar-sweetened soft drinks, diet soft drinks, and serum uric acid level: The third national health and nutrition examination survey. *Arthritis and Rheumatism, 59*(1), 109–116.

Ferdinand, K. C. (2020). Uncontrolled hypertension in sub-Saharan Africa: Now is the time to address a looming crisis. Journal of Clinical Hypertension (Greenwich), 22(11), 2111-2113. https://doi.org/10.1111/jch.14046

Feig, D. I., Soletsky, B., & Johnson, R. J. (2008). Effect of allopurinol on blood pressure of adolescents with newly diagnosed essential hypertension: A randomized trial. JAMA, 300(8), 924-932. https://doi.org/10.1001/jama.300.8.924

Feig, D. I., Madero, M., Jalal, D. I., Sanchez-Lozada, L. G., & Johnson, R. J. (2013). Uric acid and the origins of hypertension. Journal of Pediatrics, 162(5), 896-902. https://doi.org/10.1016/j.jpeds.2012.12.078

Jose, P. A., & Raj, D. (2015). Gut microbiota in hypertension. Current Opinion in Nephrology and Hypertension, 24(5), 403-409. https://doi.org/10.1097/MNH.0000000000000149"

Mager, D. E., Wan, R., Brown, M., Cheng, A., Wareski, P., Abernethy, D. R., & Mattson, M. P. (2006). Caloric restriction and intermittent fasting alter spectral measures of heart rate and blood pressure variability in rats. FASEB Journal, 20(5), 631–637. [CrossRef]

Malinowski, B., Zalewska, K., Węsierska, A., Sokołowska, M. M., Socha, M., Liczner, G., Pawlak-Osińska, K., & Wiciński, M. (2019). Intermittent fasting in cardiovascular disorders—An overview. Nutrients, 11(3), 673. https://doi.org/10.3390/nu11030673

Santisteban, M. M., Qi, Y., Zubcevic, J., Kim, S., Yang, T., Shenoy, V., Cole-Jeffrey, C. T., Lobaton, G. O., Stewart, D. C., Rubiano, A., Simmons, C. S., Garcia-Pereira, F., Johnson, R. D., Pepine, C. J., & Raizada, M. K. (2017). Hypertension-linked pathophysiological alterations in the gut. Circulation Research, 120(2), 312-323. https://doi.org/10.1161/CIRCRESAHA.116.309006

Shi, H., Zhang, B., Abo-Hamzy, T., Nelson, J. W., Ambati, C. S. R., Petrosino, J. F., Bryan, R. M. Jr, & Durgan, D. J. (2021). Restructuring the gut microbiota by intermittent fasting lowers blood pressure. Circulation Research, 128(9), 1240-1254. https://doi.org/10.1161/CIRCRESAHA.120.318155 Erratum in: Circulation Research, 130(5), e18. PMID: 33596669; PMCID: PMC8085162.

Toledo, F. W., Grundler, F., Bergouignan, A., Drinda, S., & Michalsen, A. (2019). Safety, health improvement, and well-being during a 4 to 21-day fasting period in an observational study including 1422 subjects. PLoS ONE, 14(1), e0209353. [Google Scholar]

Wang, H., Wang, A. X., Aylor, K., & Barrett, E. J. (2013). Nitric oxide directly promotes vascular endothelial insulin transport. Diabetes, 62(12), 4030–4042. https://doi.org/10.2337/db13-0627

World Health Organization. (2014, November 1). Salt - the hidden danger in the Pacific. https://www.who.int/westernpacific/about/how-we-work/pacific-support/news/detail/01-11-2014-salt-the-hidden-danger-in-the-pacific. Accessed on 21 February 2023.

World Health Organization. (2022, June 21). Dialogue with the private sector on medicines and health technologies for hypertension. https://www.who.int/news-room/events/detail/2022/06/21/default-calendar/dialogue-with-the-private-sector-on-medicines-and-health-technologies-for-hypertension--june-2022 (accessed on 20 February 2023).

Prostate health

Canadian Cancer Society. (2021). Benign prostatic hyperplasia. Last medical review February 2021. https://cancer.ca/en/cancer-information/cancer-types/prostate/what-is-prostate-cancer/benign-prostatic-hyperplasia

Chen, X., Zhao, Y., Tao, Z., et al. (2021). Coffee consumption and risk of prostate cancer: A systematic review and meta-analysis. *BMJ Open, 11*(e038902). https://doi.org/10.1136/bmjopen-2020-038902.

Ho, E., & Song, Y. (2009). Zinc and prostatic cancer. *Current Opinion in Clinical Nutrition and Metabolic Care, 12*(6), 640-645. https://doi.org/10.1097/MCO.0b013e32833106ee. PMID: 19684515; PMCID: PMC4142760.

Justin, R. G., et al. (2023). Coffee intake, caffeine metabolism genotype, and survival among men with prostate cancer. *Journal of European Urology Oncology, 3*(3), 282-288. https://euoncology.europeanurology.com/article/S2588-9311(22)00138-9/fulltext

National Cancer Institute, NIH. (2022, May 11). Prostate cancer, Nutrition, and dietary supplement, patients version. https://www.cancer.gov/about-cancer/treatment/cam/patient/prostate-supplements-pdq#:~:text=Some%20population%20studies%20in%20men,who%20do%20not%20have%20cancer

National Health Service. (2023). Overview - Benign prostate enlargement. https://www.nhs.uk/conditions/prostate-enlargement/ Last medical review 8 June 2023

Perdomo, F., Cabrera Fránquiz, F., Cabrera, J., & Serra-Majem, L. (2012). Influencia del procedimiento culinario sobre la biodisponibilidad del licopeno en el tomate [Influence of cooking procedure on the bioavailability of lycopene in tomatoes]. *Nutrición Hospitalaria, 27*(5), 1542-1546. https://doi.org/10.3305/nh.2012.27.5.5908. PMID: 23478703.

Tips to burn belly fat

Carlsson, S., Hammar, N., Grill, V., & Kaprio, J. (2003). Alcohol consumption and the incidence of type 2 diabetes: A 20-year follow-up of the Finnish twin cohort study. *Diabetes Care, 26*(10), 2785-2790. https://doi.org/10.2337/diacare.26.10.2785. PMID: 14514580.

Cullmann, M., Hilding, A., & Östenson, C. G. (2012). Alcohol consumption and risk of pre-diabetes and type 2 diabetes development in a Swedish population. *Diabetic Medicine, 29*(4), 441-452. https://doi.org/10.1111/j.1464-5491.2011.03450.x. PMID: 21916972.

Kamara, B. I., Brand, D. J., Brandt, E. V., & Joubert, E. (2004). Phenolic metabolites from honeybush tea (Cyclopia subternata). *Journal of Agricultural and Food Chemistry, 52*(17), 5391-5395. https://doi.org/10.1021/jf040097z. PMID: 15315375.

Lindtner, C., Scherer, T., Zielinski, E., Filatova, N., Fasshauer, M., Tonks, N. K., Puchowicz, M., & Buettner, C. (2013). Binge drinking induces whole-body insulin resistance by impairing hypothalamic insulin action. *Science Translational Medicine, 5*(170), 170ra14. https://doi.org/10.1126/scitranslmed.3005123. PMID: 23363978; PMCID: PMC3740748.

World Health Organization. (2013). Obesity: Health consequences of being overweight. Retrieved from https://www.who.int/news-room/questions-and-answers/item/obesity-health-consequences-of-being-overweight#:~:text=Carrying%20extra%20fat%20leads%20to,premature%20death%20and%20substantial%20disability.

Yaribeygi, H., Maleki, M., Butler, A. E., Jamialahmadi, T., & Sahebkar, A. (2022). Molecular mechanisms linking stress and insulin resistance. *EXCLI Journal, 21*, 317-334. https://doi.org/10.17179/excli2021-4382. PMID: 35368460; PMCID: PMC8971350.

Yaribeygi, H., Maleki, M., Butler, A. E., Jamialahmadi, T., & Sahebkar, A. (2022). Molecular mechanisms linking stress and insulin resistance. *EXCLI Journal, 21*, 317-334. https://doi.org/10.17179/excli2021-4382. PMID: 35368460; PMCID: PMC8971350.

You can Prevent and treat Fibroid

Brewster, L. M., Haan, Y., & van Montfrans, G. A. (2022). Cardiometabolic risk and cardiovascular disease in young women with uterine fibroids. *Cureus, 14*(10), e30740. https://doi.org/10.7759/cureus.30740

Qin H, Lin Z, Vásquez E, Luan X, Guo F, Xu L. Association between obesity and the risk of uterine fibroids: a systematic review and meta-analysis. *J Epidemiol Community Health*. 2021;75(2):197-204. doi:1136/jech-2019-213364

Calories in and out -Exercise and weight loss

Cox, C. E. (2017). Role of physical activity for weight loss and weight maintenance. *Diabetes Spectrum, 30*(3), 157-160. https://doi.org/10.2337/ds17-0013. PMID: 28848307; PMCID: PMC5556592.

Manini, T. M. (2010). Energy expenditure and aging. *Ageing Research Reviews, 9*(1), 1-11. https://doi.org/10.1016/j.arr.2009.08.002. PMID: 19698803; PMCID: PMC2818133.

Molé, P. A. (1990). Impact of energy intake and exercise on resting metabolic rate. *Sports Medicine, 10*(2), 72-87. https://doi.org/10.2165/00007256-199010020-00002. PMID: 2204100.

Most, J., & Redman, L. M. (2020). Impact of calorie restriction on energy metabolism in humans. *Experimental Gerontology, 133*, 110875. https://doi.org/10.1016/j.exger.2020.110875. PMID: 32057825; PMCID: PMC9036397.

Recipes

Barak, S., & Mudgil, D. (2014). Locust bean gum: processing, properties and food applications--a review. *International Journal of Biological Macromolecules, 66,* 74-80. https://doi.org/10.1016/j.ijbiomac.2014.02.017

Fallon, S., & Enig, M. G. (2001). *Nourishing traditions: The cookbook that challenges politically correct nutrition and the diet dictocrats* (Revised second edition).

National Academies of Sciences, Engineering, and Medicine. 2006. Lost Crops of Africa: Volume II: Vegetables. Washington, DC: The National Academies Press. https://doi.org/10.17226/11763.

The Institute for Functional Medicine. (2015). *Mito Food Plan: Weekly planner and recipes.*

The Institute for Functional Medicine. (2016). *Mito Food Plan: Comprehensive guide.*

Printed in the United States
by Baker & Taylor Publisher Services